Withholding and Withdrawing Life-prolonging Medical Treatment
Guidance for decision making

Books should be returned to the SDH Library on or before
the date stamped above unless a renewal has been arranged

Salisbury District Hospital Library
Telephone: Salisbury (01722) 336262 extn. 4432 / 33
Out of hours answer machine in operation

Withholding and Withdrawing Life-prolonging Medical Treatment

Guidance for decision making

THIRD EDITION

British Medical Association

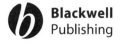

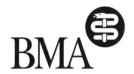

First published 1999
Second edition 2001
Third edition 2007

2   2008

ISBN: 978-1-4051-5957-9

Catalogue records for this title are available from the British Library and the Library of Congress

Set in 9.5/12 by Techbooks, India
Printed and bound in Singapore by COS Printers Pte Ltd

Commissioning Editor: Mary Banks
Editorial Assistant: Vicki Pittman
Development Editor: Charlie Hamlyn
Production Controller: Rachel Edwards

For further information on Blackwell Publishing, visit our website:
http://www.blackwellpublishing.com

The publisher's policy is to use permanent paper from mills that operate a sustainable forestry policy,
and which has been manufactured from pulp processed using acid-free and elementary chlorine-free
practices. Furthermore, the publisher ensures that the text paper and cover board used have met
acceptable environmental accreditation standards.

Contents

Medical Ethics Committee

A publication from the BMA's Medical Ethics Committee (MEC) whose membership for 2006/07 was:

Professor Parveen Kumar	President, BMA
Dr Michael Wilks*	Chairman of the Representative Body, BMA
Mr James Johnson	Chairman of Council, BMA
Dr David Pickersgill	Treasurer, BMA
Dr Anthony Calland	Chairman, Medical Ethics Committee; General Practitioner, Gwent
Dr Jonathan Brett	Junior doctor, general practice, Newcastle-upon-Tyne
Dr John Chisholm*	General Practitioner, London
Dr Peter Dangerfield	Medical Academic, Liverpool
Professor Bobbie Farsides*	Professor of Medical Law and Ethics, Brighton
Professor Ilora Finlay*	Consultant in Palliative Medicine, Cardiff
Professor Robin Gill*	Professor of Modern Theology, Canterbury
Professor Raanan Gillon*	General Practitioner; Professor of Medical Ethics, London
Dr Evan Harris*	Member of Parliament; former hospital doctor, Oxford
Professor John Harris	Sir David Alliance Professor of Bioethics, Manchester
Professor Emily Jackson*	Professor of Law, London
Dr Craig Knott	House Officer, London
Dr Surendra Kumar	General Practitioner, Widnes, Cheshire
Professor Sheila McLean*	Director of Institute of Law and Ethics, Glasgow
Professor Jonathan Montgomery	Professor of Health Care Law, Southampton
Professor Ruud ter Meulen	Professor of Ethics in Medicine, Bristol
Dr Peter Tiplady (deputy)	Retired, East Cumbria

Dr Frank Wells (deputy)	Retired, Suffolk
Dr Jan Wise	Consultant Psychiatrist, London
Dr John Jenkins	General Medical Council Observer
Ms Jane O'Brien	General Medical Council Observer
Mr Chris Chaloner	Royal College of Nursing Observer

*Sub-group of the MEC to discuss this guidance

Editorial board for the third edition

Acknowledgements for the third edition

We would like to thank those individuals and organisations who generously gave their time to review an earlier draft of this guidance. Whilst these contributions helped to inform the BMA's views, it should not be assumed that this guidance necessarily reflects the views of all those who contributed. We would particularly like to thank Anna Batchelor, Intensive Care Society; Beverley Taylor, Office of the Official Solicitor; Charlie McLaughlan, Royal College of Anaesthetists; Chris Chaloner, Royal College of Nursing; Donald Lyons, Mental Welfare Commission Scotland; Emma Wilbraham, Department of Health; Kathleen Glancy, Scottish Executive Health Department; Mike Hinchliffe, Children and Family Court Advisory and Support Service (CAFCASS); Ranald Macdonald, NHS Scotland Central Legal Office; Resuscitation Council (UK); Sandra McDonald, Office of the Public Guardian (Scotland); Sharon Burton and Roger Worthington, General Medical Council; Toby Williamson, Department for Constitutional Affairs.

Introduction

In medicine, decisions are made on a daily basis about the provision, withholding or withdrawing of treatments, some of which could prolong life. Treatments which might provide a therapeutic benefit are not inevitably given but are weighed according to a number of factors, such as the patient's wishes, the treatment's invasiveness, side-effects, limits of efficacy and the resources available. The Intensive Care Society has estimated that approximately 50,000 patients are admitted to intensive care units in England and Wales each year. Of these, 30% (15,000 patients) die without leaving hospital, most as a result of active treatment being withdrawn [1].

Although not uncommon, few issues in medicine are more complex and difficult than those addressed by patients, their relatives and their doctors concerning the decision to withhold or withdraw potentially life-prolonging treatment. Technological developments continually extend the range of treatment options available to prolong life when organ or system failure would naturally result in death. Cardiopulmonary resuscitation, renal dialysis, artificial nutrition, hydration and ventilation prolong life and, in some cases, allow time for recovery but these techniques cannot, in themselves, reverse a patient's disease. Patients with progressive conditions such as motor neurone disease can have their lives prolonged by the application of technology, but their underlying illness cannot be cured and deterioration in their condition is unavoidable. The condition of other patients, for example those with very severe brain damage, may remain stable for many years if life-prolonging treatment is provided but they may have no hope of recovering more than very minimal levels of awareness of their surroundings. They may lack the ability to interact with others or capacity for self-awareness or self-directed action. In such severely damaged patients, interventions to prolong life by artificial means may fail to provide sufficient benefit to justify the burdens of intervention (see Section 9) and the proper course of action may be to withhold or withdraw further treatment.

Most people accept that treatment should not be prolonged indefinitely when it has ceased to provide a benefit for the patient. But patients and their families, doctors and other members of the clinical team and society as a whole need reassurance that individual decisions are carefully thought through, based on the best quality information available and follow a widely agreed procedure. Decisions need to be made on an individual basis, assessing the particular circumstances, wishes and values of the patient to ensure that treatment is neither withdrawn too quickly nor unnecessarily prolonged. It is essential that there are clear, robust and transparent procedures for making these decisions. The BMA is very pleased to note that, over recent years, comprehensive guidance has been developed outlining the criteria and steps to be followed in making these decisions, particularly where difficult assessments are required about the best interests of incapacitated patients. In addition to the BMA's guidance, first published in 1999, there is now also detailed advice from the General Medical Council [2] and from the Royal College of Paediatrics and Child Health [3]. There is also statutory guidance for those providing treatment for adults who lack capacity, in the form of Codes of Practice under the Adults with Incapacity (Scotland) Act 2000 [4] and the Mental Capacity Act 2005 [5]. Nevertheless, there is only benefit in having guidance if it is available to, and used by, those responsible for making these decisions. Occasional media reporting has served to remind us that best practice is not yet universal and that we all have a responsibility to ensure that good communication and decision-making procedures are followed in all cases. In this document, the BMA seeks to provide a coherent and comprehensive set of principles which apply to all decisions to withhold or withdraw life-prolonging treatment. It is hoped that this general guidance will stimulate the development of accessible local policies and guidelines as part of a wider network of safeguards for doctors and patients.

The need for guidance in this area became clear from a wide-ranging consultation exercise undertaken by the BMA in 1998. This led to the first edition of this guidance being published in 1999. A second edition was published in 2001 to incorporate specific guidance on the impact of the Human Rights Act. This third edition includes subsequent developments in legislation – specifically the Mental Capacity Act (which at the time of writing was due to come into force in 2007) – and the common law. Although these changes have clarified some aspects of the law, some legal uncertainties remain and judicial review will still be required in particular cases. Part of the aim of this guidance is to identify the type of cases where decisions may be made by the patient, the health care team and/or those close to the patient and those where a declaration from a court is required. This guidance does not set out to give definitive legal advice but to explain the legal and ethical principles that underpin decision making in this area and to help health professionals to recognise when further advice is needed. Of course, the law will not remain static and information about any major developments following publication will be posted on the BMA's website at www.bma.org.uk/ethics.

We hope that this guidance will give confidence to those required to make these difficult decisions and the families of those on whose behalf the decisions are made. The importance of good communication at all stages of the decision-making process cannot be overstated and this forms a central part of our guidance. At the time of writing the Mental Capacity Act 2005 was scheduled to come into force in two stages – in April and September 2007. For more information on the implementation of the Act, see the BMA's website at: www.bma.org.uk/ethics.

Part 1 **How to use this guidance**

1. Scope, purpose and structure of this guidance

1.1. This document covers a wide range of different scenarios, treatments, patients and UK jurisdictions. With this in mind some parts of the guidance cover the general moral, legal and practical issues that apply to all decisions while other sections provide more specific information enabling readers to quickly identify the information they need.

We recommend that Parts 2, 3 and 4 of this guidance be read first as they set the scene for decision making, define the concepts and definitions used throughout and address the practical considerations that apply to all decisions. From Part 5 onwards the guidance is divided up into sections based on whether the patient is an adult who has or lacks capacity or a child or young person who has or lacks capacity. Clearly there is overlap and some repetition is inevitable but cross-referencing is used wherever possible. Although we have tried to give a clear indication of the important factors to consider with each type of patient, information that is provided in other sections may also be helpful in giving an overall picture of the decision-making process.

Summary boxes have been included throughout the text to ease navigation through the guidance and legal cases are summarised to illustrate the relevant legal points. Although some of these cases are now quite old and were decided before the Human Rights Act and mental capacity legislation came into force, they remain important in guiding both legal and medical practice.

This guidance is intended to complement, and not replace, statutory guidance issued under mental capacity legislation. It is essential that all health professionals, who are working in England, Wales and Scotland with adults who lack capacity, are familiar with the statutory Codes of Practice published under the Mental Capacity Act 2005 and the Adults with Incapacity (Scotland) Act 2000.

1.2. The main focus of this guidance is decisions to withdraw or withhold life-prolonging treatment from patients who are likely to live for weeks, months or possibly years, if treatment is provided but who, without treatment, will or may die earlier. In some areas mention is also made of treatment decisions for those patients whose imminent death is inevitable.

This guidance focuses on the process through which decisions are made to withdraw or withhold life-prolonging treatment from all types of patients – adults with capacity, adults lacking capacity, young people with capacity and children and young people who lack capacity. Such decisions are taken on a regular basis, throughout the country where, for example, patients with capacity decide that, for them, the burdens of further aggressive chemotherapy or dialysis outweigh the potential benefits. Or, where patients lack capacity, it is judged that invasive treatment would not be in their best interests because it is unable to provide a level of recovery that would justify the intervention. Similarly, a decision may be made that, in the event of cardiac arrest, a patient should not be subjected to cardiopulmonary resuscitation because the chances of recovery, or the level of recovery that could reasonably be expected, would not provide a net benefit to that patient. These decisions are always profound and cannot be taken lightly. The intention of this guidance is to set down established good practice in this area to help all those involved with making such decisions.

1.3. This document is not an attempt to define rules which must be followed. Rather, it provides general guidance about the principles and factors to take into account in reaching a decision.

This guidance does not provide a simple set of instructions to be followed without reflection but a tool to inform and aid decision making; it does not provide easy answers but offers an approach through which an appropriate decision may be reached. It reflects the standards that doctors must meet, as required by law and set out by the General Medical Council, and sets these standards within a broader context with a view to providing practical advice for decision making. Although principally aimed at health professionals, others who are responsible for decision making, such as the parents of young children and those who are appointed as personal welfare attorneys or deputies for incapacitated adults, may also find this guidance useful. This document provides a basis for discussion between all those involved in making decisions, which will include health professionals, the patient and those close to or representing the patient.

Part 2 **Defining key terms and concepts**

This section defines some of the key terms and concepts that are used throughout this document. It is useful to read through this section to provide general information about, and set the scene for, decision making before moving on to the more specific information provided in later sections. In order to minimise repetition these definitions are not repeated later in the text and so it is also necessary to refer back to these definitions when reading later sections of the guidance.

2. The primary goal of medicine

2.1. The primary goal of medical treatment is to benefit the patient by restoring or maintaining the patient's health as far as possible, maximising benefit and minimising harm. If a patient with capacity has refused the treatment or if the patient lacks capacity and the treatment would fail or ceases to provide a net benefit to the patient, then that goal cannot be realised and the treatment should, ethically and legally, be withheld or withdrawn. Good quality care and palliation of symptoms should, however, continue.

Health care is normally based on the common sense assumption that life-prolonging treatment is beneficial and that most patients would want it. In the majority of cases, therefore, it is provided unless the patient refuses it or the patient's death is imminent and inevitable. There are, however, some extreme cases where life-prolonging treatment fails to provide a net benefit to the patient because it is unable to achieve a level of recovery that justifies the corresponding burdens of the treatment. Or, the treatment may keep the patient alive but be unable to stop the progression of the disease or provide any hope of the patient recovering self-awareness, awareness of others and the ability to intentionally interact with them (see Section 9). Patients sometimes decide that the stage has been reached beyond which, for them, continued treatment aimed at prolonging life, although possible, would be inappropriate. Where patients lack capacity, these decisions must be taken in a way that reflects their wishes or, if these are not known, their best interests. This may include a decision not to provide or continue to provide an intervention which is not of benefit to the patient even if the withholding or withdrawing of that treatment allows the patient to die earlier than if the treatment were provided or continued.

2.2. Prolonging a patient's life usually, but not always, provides a benefit to that patient. Although the courts have emphasised that there is a strong presumption in favour of providing life-prolonging treatment, it is not an appropriate goal of medicine to prolong life at all costs, with no regard to its quality or the burdens of treatment.

High regard for the value of life does not necessarily imply a duty to always give life-prolonging treatment. It is not the case that all lives must be prolonged by artificial means for as long as technically possible. Nor is this what most people would want. The aim is to reach a decision about the provision of treatment that is right for that particular individual, based on his or her clinical condition and personal situation. The guiding principles that underpin these difficult judgements are that such decisions must protect the dignity, comfort and rights of the patient and take into account the wishes, if known, of the patient and, where the patient lacks capacity, the views of those close to the patient.

2.3. Developments in technology have led to a misperception in society that death can almost always be postponed. There needs to be a recognition that there comes a point in all lives where no more can reasonably or helpfully be done to benefit patients other than keeping them comfortable and free from pain.

With life-prolonging treatment some patients could potentially survive for many years without achieving awareness or being able to interact with others. This has led to unrealistic expectations in society about the extent to which it is possible to postpone death such that death is sometimes seen not as a natural, inevitable event but as a failure of medicine. Doctors should strive to assist patients to understand that life cannot be prolonged indefinitely and to accept the inevitability of death. It is only with this acceptance that people will feel able to plan in advance and state clearly their wishes for end-of-life care. Many patients retain capacity and are able to make their own decisions until very close to the end of their lives but for those who lose capacity decisions need to be made on their behalf that reflect their wishes, hopes and aspirations. This task is much easier if people give thought to what they would want while they have capacity and make their views known to their family or appointed attorney and health care team.

3. Life-prolonging treatment

3.1. Life-prolonging treatment refers to all treatments or procedures that have the potential to postpone the patient's death and includes cardiopulmonary resuscitation, artificial ventilation, specialised treatments for particular conditions such as chemotherapy or dialysis, antibiotics when given for a potentially life-threatening infection and artificial nutrition and hydration.

Developments in technology mean that patients can increasingly be kept alive when previously their condition would inevitably have resulted in early death. This means that the basic biological functions can be maintained, artificially, in many patients even though there may be no prospect of the patient recovering or developing any awareness of his or her surroundings.

4. Capacity and incapacity

4.1. Patients over 16 years of age are presumed to have the capacity to make decisions for themselves unless the contrary is proven. Where there is doubt about whether an individual has the capacity to make the decision in question, further enquiries should be made.

The fact that an individual has made a decision that appears to others to be irrational or unjustified should not necessarily be taken as evidence of lack of capacity although it would raise questions about whether that person has understood the implications of their choice and further discussion might be needed. It is also inappropriate to make assumptions about lack of capacity based merely on individuals' age, appearance or aspects of their behaviour. Individuals are, however, considered legally unable to make decisions for themselves where they are unable to:
• understand the information relevant to the decision;
• retain that information;
• use or weigh that information as part of the process of making the decision; or
• communicate the decision (whether by talking, using sign language or other means) [6].
   An individual should not be deemed to lack capacity unless efforts have been made to maximise the patient's decision-making capacity.
   The test for capacity is task specific – whether somebody has capacity to do something depends on what that something is – and so for all patients the complexity of the decision needs to be considered as part of the assessment. For example, the level of capacity required to take a relatively straightforward

decision about whether to have a broken arm set is not as great as that required to decide whether or not to have chemotherapy where the treatment is far more complex and chances of success are less than optimal. In addition, English courts have held that the implications of the decision are also relevant factors to consider and have stated that the graver the consequences of the decision, the commensurately greater the level of capacity required to take that decision. This point has not been made by courts in other parts of the UK and the reasoning behind this statement has been questioned. It has, for example, been argued that the test for capacity should relate to the individual's *ability* to make the decision in question and that should be independent of the outcome of the decision [7]. The practical point for doctors, however, is that when assessing individuals' mental capacity to choose a course of action that is likely to have detrimental consequences for their health, such as refusing life-prolonging treatment, there should be more evidence that patients fulfil the four criteria stated above than for other decisions with less serious consequences.

Further information about capacity and incapacity can be found in the mental capacity legislation codes of practice.

5. Duty of care

5.1. A fundamental part of the health care team's positive duty of care is to take reasonable steps (see Section 17) to keep the patient alive, where that is the patient's known wish. The only exceptions to this general duty would be if patients with capacity refused the treatment or if patients lacked capacity and it was not considered in their best interests to be kept alive artificially (see Section 9).

In the case of Burke v. General Medical Council (GMC) the Court of Appeal stated that where a patient with capacity requests artificial nutrition and hydration this must be provided [8]. The Court was careful to explain that this did not mean that patients had the right to demand particular forms of treatment but rather that a fundamental aspect of the duty of care is to take reasonable steps to keep the patient alive where that is the patient's known wish. This raises a question about what is 'reasonable' which needs to be considered in the context of each case bearing in mind the need to balance the competing clinical and resource needs of different patients (see Section 17).

Burke v. GMC

Mr Oliver Leslie Burke was a 45-year-old man with cerebellar ataxia with peripheral neuropathy, a progressively degenerative condition that follows a similar course to multiple sclerosis. As his condition worsened he would lose the ability to swallow, requiring artificial nutrition and hydration (ANH). Medical evidence indicated that he would retain mental capacity until very close to his death.

Mr Burke was concerned that the GMC's guidance on withholding and withdrawing life-prolonging treatment gave doctors the discretion to decide whether ANH should be provided and allowed them to withdraw ANH even if his death was not imminent. He challenged the guidance, claiming that it was incompatible with the Human Rights Act.

In July 2004 Mr Justice Munby upheld the challenge, ruling that some parts of the GMC's guidance were not compatible with the Human Rights Act. This decision was, however, overturned by the Court of Appeal. The Court of Appeal made clear that there was never any question of ANH being withdrawn before the final stages of Mr Burke's disease and that he did not need to go to court to ensure this. This is because he had always made it clear that he would want to receive this treatment when his health deteriorated and when he was no longer able to express his wishes. The Court of Appeal held that 'autonomy and the right to self-determination do not entitle the patient to insist on receiving a particular medical treatment regardless of the nature of the treatment. In so far as a doctor has a legal obligation to provide treatment this cannot be founded simply upon the fact that the patient demands it'. Explaining the relationship between a doctor's duty of care and a patient's request for treatment, the judge said: 'Where ANH is necessary to keep the patient alive, the duty of care will normally require the doctors to supply ANH . . . Where the competent patient makes it plain that he or she wishes to be kept alive by ANH . . . the patient's wish will merely underscore that duty'. The Court of Appeal emphasised that to deliberately interrupt life-prolonging treatment, in the face of a patient's expressed wish to be kept alive, with the intention of thereby terminating the patient's life, would leave the doctor with no answer to a charge of murder.

Mr Burke was denied leave to appeal to the House of Lords and his application to the European Court of Human Rights was rejected.

R (on the application of Burke) v. *GMC* [9]

The duty to provide life-prolonging treatment, where this is the patient's wish, does not extend to the provision of treatment that is not clinically indicated. The Court of Appeal endorsed the following principles that had been put forward by the GMC:

- the doctor decides what treatment options would provide overall clinical benefit for the patient;
- these options are offered to the patient, explaining the benefits, risks and side-effects of each;
- the patient decides which, if any, of the treatment options he or she wishes to accept;
- if one option is accepted, the doctor will provide it; and

• if the patient refuses all the options and requests an alternative which was not offered, the doctor will discuss that treatment with him or her. The doctor is not, however, obliged to offer that treatment if he or she does not believe it to be clinically indicated, although a second opinion should be offered [10].

Where patients lack capacity and have not made a valid advance decision (see Sections 28 and 32), the duty of care requires action to be taken that is in the patients' best interests (see Sections 9 and 40).

6. Quality of life

6.1.   Terms such as 'quality of life' can be problematic and ambiguous. But whether articulated or not, the concept of 'quality of life' is unavoidable when discussing the provision of life-prolonging treatment. The courts have specifically stated that the quality of life which could reasonably be expected following treatment is an appropriate factor to take into account when making treatment decisions.

Patients generally have strong views about what would be an acceptable quality of life for themselves and most are able to make their own decisions about whether to accept the treatments offered. When used by others in relation to people lacking capacity, however, the term can be interpreted to imply that some people's lives are less valued. Despite this inherent difficulty with the concept, its use is unavoidable. A vital part of the treatment decision rests on the issue of whether the proposed measures can restore patients to a way of living they would be likely to consider acceptable, despite any side-effects or disadvantages of treatment. Nevertheless, it must always be clear that the doctor's role is not to assess the value or worth of the patient's life but rather the value of the treatment for the patient. Care must be taken to avoid making unjustifiable assumptions about best interests (see Section 19) and to ensure the decision relates to what the *patient* would find acceptable, not what the decision maker would find acceptable. Wherever possible, discussion should take place with those close to or representing patients who lack capacity as part of the assessment of best interests. If, after consultation and discussion, it is agreed that the treatment is unable to benefit the patient, in terms of restoring that person's health to a level that he or she would find acceptable, its use must be open to question.

The acceptability of taking account of the patient's quality of life in making treatment decisions was confirmed by the High Court in 1996. In that case, the decision to withhold life-prolonging treatment from a patient, R [11], who was born with a serious malformation of the brain as well as cerebral palsy, was challenged on the grounds that it was 'irrational and unlawful' to permit medical treatment to be withheld on the basis of an assessment of a patient's quality of life. The case was dismissed. Sir Stephen Brown said that the same principles applied for adults as for babies, as set out by Lord Justice Taylor in Re J who said:

'I consider the correct approach is for the Court to judge the quality of life the child would have to endure if given the treatment and decide whether in all the circumstances such a life would be so afflicted as to be intolerable.'

Taylor LJ went on to say:

'The test must be whether the child in question, if capable of exercising sound judgment, would consider the life tolerable. . . . [This approach] takes account of the strong instinct to preserve one's life even in circumstances which an outsider, not himself at risk of death, might consider unacceptable. The circumstances to be considered would, in appropriate cases, include the degree of existing disability and any additional suffering or aggravation of the disability which the treatment itself would superimpose. In an accident case, as opposed to one involving disablement from birth, the child's pre-accident quality of life and its perception of what has been lost may also be factors relevant to whether the residual life would be intolerable to that child.' [12]

Re R

R was born in 1972 with a serious malformation of the brain and cerebral palsy and developed severe epilepsy at the age of 8. At the age of 23 he had not developed any formal means of communication, was unable to walk or sit upright unaided, he was believed to be blind and deaf, was incontinent and, being unable to chew, was fed by having food syringed to the back of his mouth. The only response to touch appeared to be when he was cuddled when he gave an indication of pleasure. Although not in a persistent vegetative state he was believed to exist in a 'low awareness state'.

In 1995 R was admitted to hospital on five occasions with life-threatening episodes and treatment was provided. After the fifth admission and following discussion with R's parents it was agreed that in any future cardiac arrest, cardiopulmonary resuscitation would not be started (i.e. a do not attempt resuscitation order – DNAR). The DNAR was, however, opposed by staff at the day care centre that R attended and a judicial review of the decision was sought on

> the grounds that it was 'irrational and unlawful' to permit medical treatment to be withheld on the basis of an assessment of a patient's quality of life. The Court rejected this argument, relying on the 1990 case of Re J in which the Court decided that it was appropriate to consider whether the patient's life, if treatment was given, would be 'so afflicted as to be intolerable'. The Court agreed that no attempt should be made to resuscitate R in the event of a cardiac arrest.
>
> Re R (*Adult: Medical Treatment*) [13]

Quality of life assessment tools [14] are important for research and for monitoring an individual patient's response to therapy, but they are generally too limited in scope and domains covered to form a basis for individual clinical decision making when best interests decisions are to be taken.

7. Benefit

7.1. Health professionals have a general duty to provide treatment which benefits their patients. Benefit, in this context, has its ordinary meaning of an advantage or net gain for the patient but is broader than simply whether the treatment achieves a particular physiological goal. It includes both medical and other, less tangible, benefits.

The provision of treatment to prolong life is usually but not always a benefit. Benefit accrues not only when progress can be made or recovery achieved; in some cases patients benefit from treatment that is able to maintain the status quo and prevent further deterioration. In other cases, the treatment may keep the patient alive but be unable to stop the progression of the disease or provide any hope of the person achieving any level of self-awareness or awareness of others and the ability to intentionally interact with them (see Section 9). In these most extreme cases of profound disability, the burdens of providing treatment to prolong life may outweigh the potential benefits and, in such cases, attention should shift to providing all aspects of good quality end-of-life care. In deciding which treatment should be offered, the expectation must be that the advantages outweigh the drawbacks for the individual patient. Where patients have capacity they are in the best position to judge what represents an acceptable level of burden or risk for them. If patients with capacity refuse life-prolonging treatment, their wishes must be respected even if the health care team believes that treatment would be beneficial.

The Court of Appeal confirmed in 2005 that 'where life depends upon the continued provision of [artificial nutrition and hydration] there can be no question of the supply of ANH not being clinically indicated unless a clinical decision has been taken that the life in question should come to an end. That is not a decision that can lawfully be taken in the case of a competent patient who expresses the wish to remain alive' [15].

Where patients lack capacity, their known previously expressed wishes should form a core part of assessing the benefit to them of providing life-prolonging treatment. If the patient is known to have held the view that there is intrinsic value in being alive, irrespective of the quality of that life, then life-prolonging treatment would, in virtually all cases, provide a net benefit for that particular individual. Many people, however, do not take that view. The vast majority of people with, even very severe, physical or mental disabilities are able to experience and gain pleasure from some aspects of their lives. Where, however, the disability is so profound that individuals have no or minimal levels of awareness of their own existence and no hope of recovering awareness, or where they experience severe untreatable pain or other distress, the question arises as to whether continuing to provide treatment aimed at prolonging that life artificially would provide a benefit to them (see Section 9). An important factor which is often considered in making these decisions is whether patients are thought to be aware of their environment or own existence as demonstrated by, for example:

• being able to interact with others;
• being aware of their own existence and having an ability to take pleasure in the fact of that existence; or
• having the ability to achieve some purposeful or self-directed action or to achieve some goal of importance to him or herself.

If treatment is unable to recover or maintain any of these abilities, this is likely to indicate that its continued provision will not be a benefit to the patient. If any one of these abilities can be achieved, then life-prolonging treatment may be of benefit and it is important to consider these factors within the context of the individual's own wishes and values where these are known, in order to assess whether the patient would, or could reasonably be expected to, consider life-prolonging treatment to be beneficial.

8. Harm

8.1. Patients may be harmed both by the withdrawal of treatment too quickly and by prolonging treatment beyond the point where it is able to benefit the patient. Patients with capacity, or patients whose views are known, are also harmed by treatment being provided or withdrawn against their wishes.

Patients with capacity are the best judge of what would be a harm or a benefit for them. Where patients are known to have refused treatment or to have clear views about the quality of life that they would find acceptable, these should be respected. To do something to individuals against their wishes can, in itself, be a harm and risks also being viewed by the courts as an infringement of their basic rights (see Section 18) and possibly a criminal offence and the tort of battery. Jehovah's Witnesses who have refused a life-prolonging blood transfusion, for example, are harmed by being given a transfusion against their stated wishes even though that may save their life. Patients do not have the right to demand treatments that are clinically inappropriate but if there is evidence that the individual would view a particular procedure as offering benefit, that view should be taken into account (see Section 26.3). Judgements should be made according to the strength of evidence available.

Where patients lack capacity, decisions to withdraw treatment that will inevitably or very probably result in a patient's death, although difficult, can be an important part of good medical care. Anecdotal reports of health professionals' reluctance to make these decisions, resulting in inappropriate admission to intensive care units and the use of invasive and, what some would consider, undignified treatment, are an example of where failing to take a decision could harm the patient. Many people, particularly elderly patients, do not want to die in hospital being subjected to invasive treatment and would rather die peacefully in their own home or surrounded by their family [16]. Patients lacking capacity are also harmed by being denied life-prolonging treatment that could provide a benefit for them. Where there is doubt about whether life-prolonging treatment would be beneficial for a particular patient, a trial of treatment, with a subsequent review, allows time for the patient's condition to stabilise and for more information to be gained about the likelihood and extent of any improvement (see Section 24.6). Failing to give patients this opportunity for improvement where it could be successful may of itself be a harm.

9. Best interests

9.1. Where patients lack capacity to make decisions for themselves, the test that must be applied to determine whether treatment should be provided is 'best interests'. This is broader than medical interests and includes the patient's own wishes and values.

'Best interests' presents an apparently reassuring standard by which decisions should be made but can be interpreted in many ways. In the past, best interests were often seen solely in terms of best medical interests, and the prolongation of life at almost any cost was often regarded as being in the patient's interests. Modern technology and the ability to sustain some essential functions far beyond the irrevocable loss of awareness and ability to interact with others increasingly demonstrate this to be unsustainable. Legal judgments about the withdrawal of life-prolonging treatment have now made clear that, in some circumstances, invasive prolongation of life need not be provided, because either it can be perceived as a harm or it would not achieve its therapeutic goal of clinical improvement (see Section 2).

The Mental Capacity Act requires that any decision relating to a patient who lacks capacity in England and Wales must be in his or her best interests. In assessing best interests account must be taken of:

- the person's past and present wishes and feelings (and, in particular, any relevant written statement made by the patient before capacity was lost);
- the beliefs and values that would be likely to influence the decision if the patient had capacity; and
- the other factors the patient would be likely to consider if able to do so [17].

Although it is usually in the best interests of patients who lack capacity to provide life-prolonging treatment, this is not always the case. The type of factors that should be taken into account in assessing whether the provision of life-prolonging treatment would be in the patient's best interests include:

- the patient's own wishes and values (where these can be ascertained) including any written statements made when the patient had capacity;
- clinical judgement about the effectiveness of the proposed treatment;
- the likelihood of the patient experiencing severe unmanageable pain or suffering;
- the level of awareness patients have of their existence and surroundings as demonstrated by, for example:
  - an ability to interact with others, however expressed;
  - capacity for self-directed action or ability to take control of any aspect of his or her life;
- the likelihood and extent of any degree of improvement in the patient's condition if treatment is provided;
- whether the invasiveness of the treatment is justified in the circumstances;
- the views of the parents, if the patient is a child;
- the views of any appointed health care proxy, welfare attorney or patient advocate;
- the views of people close to the patient, especially close relatives, partners and carers, about what the patient is likely to see as beneficial.

The UK courts have rejected 'substituted judgement' as the criterion for decision making for adults who lack capacity (whereby the decision is that which the individual is likely to have made if in a position to do so), preferring to use a supposedly more objective assessment of 'best interests'. In practice, however, part of the assessment of best interests relies on some aspects of substituted judgement. When seeking views from relatives the decision maker is trying to ascertain whether the patient would consider the benefits of treatment to outweigh the burdens, including whether the quality of life that could be achieved with treatment would be acceptable to the patient.

The Court of Appeal in the case of Mr Burke (see Section 5) referred to cases where 'life involves an extreme degree of pain, discomfort or indignity to a patient, who is sentient but not competent and who has manifested no wish to be kept alive' as being the type of cases where the courts have accepted that it may not be in the best interests of a patient lacking capacity to be kept alive artificially [18].

It is important to note that the courts have made clear, when making best interests judgements, that the decision must be that which is in the best interests of the particular patient – taking account of all relevant factors – and not that which merely represents a reasonable treatment option for patients in this position. The decision about best interests involves two steps:

1. the treatment must comply with the 'Bolam test' as amended [19] (i.e. it must be in accordance with the logical views of a responsible body of medical opinion); and
2. the decision must be in the best interests of the particular patient.

While many different courses of action would comply with the amended Bolam test, logically the best interests test should give only one answer – that which is the best available option for the patient at the time the decision is taken [20].

Additional information about assessing best interests can be found in the Mental Capacity Act Code of Practice.

10. Futility

10.1. Treatment is usually considered unable to produce the desired benefit either because it cannot achieve its physiological aim or because the burdens of the treatment are considered to outweigh the benefits for the particular individual. This is sometimes called 'futile' treatment, although this concept is problematic precisely because it combines these two different scenarios. Whilst the former is clearly a medical decision, the latter must involve consultation with patients or their relatives or advocate where this is possible within the time available.

Where treatment is of no clinical benefit and so is not clinically indicated, this is clearly a medical decision but when treatment is considered futile because it is unable to provide an acceptable quality of life, the competent patient's own view about the acceptable level of burden or risk must carry considerable weight. Treatment may be able to prolong life only for a short period and so might be considered futile but, for that particular individual, there may be benefit in having that extra time that outweighs any burdens or risks associated with the treatment (see Section 9). It is highly questionable whether a treatment could be considered to be of no 'benefit' to the patient – given a broad definition of benefit – if the patient knows, and has accepted, the chance, level and length of expected recovery and wishes to accept treatment on that basis. Where patients are not competent, those close to them and any appointed welfare attorney, deputy or advocate should be consulted before deciding that the patient's quality of life is so poor that treatment to prolong that life would be futile.

11. Basic care

11.1. The performance of procedures that are solely or primarily designed to provide comfort to the patient or alleviate that person's symptoms or distress are facets of basic care. This includes warmth, shelter, hygiene measures (such as the management of incontinence), the offer of oral nutrition and hydration and the provision of analgesia.

Whilst treatment may, in some circumstances, be withheld or withdrawn, appropriate basic care should always be provided unless actively resisted by the patient. This does not mean that all facets of basic care must be provided in all cases and refusals of basic care by patients with capacity should be respected, although it should continue to be offered. Where, however, the individual is unable to express preferences, procedures that are essential to keep the patient comfortable should be provided. If there is doubt about a patient's comfort, the presumption should be in favour of providing relief from symptoms and distress and enhancing the patient's dignity.

12. Artificial nutrition and hydration

12.1. Artificial nutrition and hydration (ANH) refers specifically to those techniques for providing nutrition or hydration that are used to bypass an inability to swallow. It includes the use of a nasogastric tube, percutaneous endoscopic gastrostomy (PEG feeding) and total parenteral nutrition [21].

Whilst the term 'artificial nutrition and hydration' is used in this guidance, it is recognised that neither the nutrition nor the hydration is, in fact, *artificial* although the methods for delivering them are. Some people prefer to use terms such as 'tube feeding' or 'technologically delivered feeding'. Since artificial nutrition and hydration has become a widely used and accepted term, however, this terminology has been used throughout this document.

Non-provision of ANH is a controversial area where views differ. Some people regard their provision as basic care which should always be provided unless the patient's imminent death is inevitable. Others make a distinction between the insertion of a feeding tube – which is classed as treatment – and the provision of nutrition and hydration through the tube, which is considered basic care [22]. From this perspective, decisions not to insert a feeding tube, or not to reinsert it if it becomes dislodged, would be legitimate medical decisions whereas a decision to stop providing nutrition and hydration through an existing tube would not. There is, however, no such distinction in the law (see Section 15). The provision of nutrition and hydration by artificial means requires the use of medical or nursing skills to overcome an inability to swallow, in the same way that the artificial provision of insulin is given to diabetic patients to overcome the body's own inability to produce that substance.

Although we refer in this guidance to artificial nutrition *and* hydration, there are good clinical reasons why hydration and nutrition should be assessed separately. For example, with some terminally ill patients subcutaneous or intravenous fluids may avoid dehydration, decrease pressure sore risk and aid comfort, but the provision of nutrition artificially would be too invasive to be in a patient's best interests. With other patients it is appropriate for both nutrition and hydration to be provided, withheld or withdrawn.

12.2. Following legal judgments, ANH are classed as medical treatments which may be withdrawn in some circumstances. The GMC requires doctors to seek a second clinical opinion before withholding or withdrawing artificial nutrition or hydration from patients whose death is not imminent [23].

Whether ANH constitutes medical treatment or basic care was one of the central questions considered by the House of Lords in the case of Tony Bland [24].

Tony Bland

Tony Bland was 17 years old when he was involved in the Hillsborough football stadium disaster in April 1989. As a result, his lungs were crushed and punctured and the supply of oxygen to his brain was interrupted. He suffered catastrophic and irreversible damage to the higher centres of the brain, leaving him in a persistent vegetative state. He could breathe unaided, but had no cognitive function. He was unable to see, hear, taste, smell, speak, or communicate in any way or feel pain. Being unable to swallow, he was fed artificially by a nasogastric tube. In 1992 an application was submitted to the court for a declaration that it would be lawful to withdraw all life-sustaining treatment, including ANH. The application had the support of Tony Bland's family, the consultant in charge of his care and two independent doctors.

In approving the application the House of Lords was satisfied that there was no therapeutic, medical or other benefit to Tony Bland in continuing to maintain his nutrition and hydration by artificial means. It was also held that the provision of artificial feeding by means of a nasogastric tube was 'medical treatment'. The view of three of the five Law Lords who considered this case was expressed by Lord Goff as follows:

> *'There is overwhelming evidence that, in the medical profession, artificial feeding is regarded as a form of medical treatment; and even if it is not strictly medical treatment, it must form part of the medical care of the patient.'*

> *Airedale NHS Trust* v. *Bland* [25]

This classification of ANH as medical treatment, which has been the published view of the BMA since 1992, has been adopted in other subsequent cases in England [26] and Scotland [27] and is now established common law.

The GMC's guidance, which is binding on all doctors, requires that a second clinical opinion is sought before artificial nutrition or hydration is withheld or withdrawn from a patient who is not imminently dying. This opinion should be sought from a senior clinician (medical or nursing) who has experience of the patient's condition and who is not directly involved in the patient's care [28]. This is to ensure that, in this most sensitive area, the patient's interests have been thoroughly considered and to provide reassurance to those close to patients and the wider public.

Mechanisms should be in place to identify all cases in which artificial nutrition and/or hydration was withheld or withdrawn from patients who were unable to swallow and who were not imminently dying. These cases should be reviewed, at a local level, in order to ensure that appropriate procedures and guidelines were followed.

12.3. In England, Wales and Northern Ireland where the patient is in a persistent vegetative state (pvs), or in a state of very low awareness closely resembling pvs, and is not imminently dying, the withdrawal of ANH currently requires legal review (see Section 30).

13. Oral nutrition and hydration

13.1. Where nutrition and hydration are provided by ordinary means – such as by cup, spoon or any other method for delivering food or nutritional supplements into the patient's mouth – or the moistening of a patient's mouth for comfort, this forms part of basic care and should not be withdrawn.

13.2. Food or water to be given by these means should always be offered but should not be forced upon patients who resist or express a clear refusal. It should also not be forced upon patients for whom the process of feeding produces an unacceptable level of burden, such as where it is likely to cause choking or aspiration of the food or fluid. Where oral feeding is unable to meet the nutritional needs of the patient, formal consideration should be given to whether artificial nutrition and/or hydration should be provided (see Section 12).

Many patients, such as babies, young children and people with disability, may require assistance with feeding but retain the ability to swallow if the food is placed in their mouth; this forms part of basic care. Evidence suggests that when patients are close to death, however, they seldom want nutrition and/or hydration and its provision may, in fact, exacerbate discomfort and suffering [29]. Good practice must, however, include good oral care to avoid the discomfort of a dry mouth.

14. Foresight and intention

14.1. Although the health care team may foresee that withholding or withdrawing life-prolonging treatment will result in the patient's death, this is fundamentally different from action taken with the purpose or objective of ending the patient's life.

Some people have argued that a doctor deciding to withhold or withdraw life-prolonging treatment (including, but not only, ANH) which will inevitably or very probably result in the patient's death must be doing so with the purpose or objective of ending that person's life. It has also been argued that a decision to withdraw medical treatment that could prolong life necessarily involves a judgement that the patient's life is not worth living. This does not, however, reflect the reality of clinical practice and nor does it represent the law. A doctor may withhold or withdraw life-prolonging treatment if the purpose of doing so is to withdraw treatment which is not a benefit to the patient and is therefore not in the patient's best interests. The emphasis here is not on the value of the patient's life but on the justification, or otherwise, for providing treatment that has the effect of prolonging the patient's life artificially.

In law, a doctor may foresee – be able to predict – that the patient will die if treatment is not provided but this must not be the sole reason for withholding it; the overriding purpose or objective must be to ensure that treatment which is not in the best interests of the patient is avoided [30]. It is only when this condition is satisfied that withholding or withdrawing treatment without the patient's consent is lawful. In other words, it is only lawful to withhold or withdraw treatment when to continue it is not in the patient's best interests. The courts have confirmed that, in such circumstances, the health team would not be in breach of its duty to protect life under the Human Rights Act (see Section 18) [31].

This distinction between foresight and intention is well established in law and is crucial to good practice since it means that doctors are not obliged to prolong life for as long as technically possible irrespective of the circumstances and the wishes of the patient. Clearly, however, these decisions are difficult and must be open, transparent and subject to scrutiny.

15. Withholding or withdrawing treatment

15.1. Although psychologically it may be easier to withhold treatment than to withdraw that which has been started, there are no necessary legal or morally relevant differences between the two actions.

The primary aim of instituting medical treatment is to provide a health benefit to the patient. The same justification is required for continuing treatment that has already been started. In fact, withdrawal of life-prolonging treatment is often morally safer than withholding it. In many cases the possibility of beneficial effects of such treatment makes it inappropriate to withhold treatment. Treatment is, therefore, often initiated in order to ascertain whether or not it is able to benefit the patient, even though it may subsequently be withdrawn when more information is available and lack of benefit is established.

The legal and moral equivalence of withholding and withdrawing treatment was expressed by Lord Goff and Lord Lowry in the Bland case (see Section 12), with the latter saying:

> 'I do not believe that there is a valid distinction between the omission to treat a patient and the abandonment of treatment which has been commenced, since to recognise such a distinction could quite illogically confer on a doctor who had refrained from treatment an immunity which did not benefit a doctor who had embarked on treatment in order to see whether it might help the patient and had abandoned the treatment when it was seen not to do so.' [32]

Although there may be no necessary legal or moral difference between withholding and withdrawing treatment when making decisions about an individual patient, this is not to say that psychologically the two are equivalent. Some people feel a significant difference in the message conveyed by withholding as opposed to withdrawing treatment. There can be an impression attached to a decision to withdraw treatment which can be interpreted as abandonment or 'giving up on the patient'; conversely, without a therapeutic trial of a treatment there can be a feeling that the patient has been denied the chance of improvement.

15.2. Treatment should never be withheld when there is a possibility that it will benefit the patient, simply because withholding is considered to be easier than any subsequent withdrawal of treatment.

There is a risk that the perceived psychological difficulty of withdrawing treatment could lead to some patients failing to receive treatment that could benefit them. Where there is uncertainty about the benefit of a particular treatment, health professionals should not be reluctant to start treatment because of the mistaken belief that, once initiated, the treatment cannot be withdrawn.

16. Conscientious objection

16.1. With very limited exceptions, doctors are not obliged to provide care to a patient that goes against their conscience or their clinical judgement. Health professionals are also not obliged to give treatment which, in their view, is contrary to the best interests of a patient who lacks capacity.

The courts have made clear on many occasions that doctors are not obliged to provide treatment contrary to their clinical judgement [33] or their conscience [34]. Where this situation arises, it is sufficient for the doctor to hand over care to a colleague. One exception to this rule is where the situation is an emergency and a termination of pregnancy is immediately necessary to save the life of the patient. In that case doctors who oppose abortion would be obliged to act contrary to their conscience. Also, in the very limited circumstances addressed in the case of Mr Burke (see Section 5) the Court of Appeal made clear that doctors would themselves be obliged to provide ANH where that was keeping a patient with capacity alive in line with his or her express wishes [35]. This exception is unlikely to have any impact on practice, however, since no doctor could argue that it was an affront to his or her conscience to provide ANH to prolong the life of a patient who had capacity and wished to stay alive.

Doctors are not obliged to provide treatment at the request of the relatives of a patient lacking capacity although where there is disagreement about whether treatment would be in the best interests of the patient it would be good practice to offer a second opinion and, in some cases, such as where the patient is a child and the parents have not given consent, it will be necessary to seek a court declaration (see Section 47.8). Where the doctor disagrees with an appointed welfare attorney or deputy about the best interests of the patient, there are established procedures to be followed (see Sections 27.3 and 31.3).

16.2. People who have a conscientious objection to withholding or withdrawing life-prolonging treatment should, wherever possible, be permitted to hand over care of the patient to a colleague.

Some people have a fundamental objection to the withholding or withdrawal of treatment or particular types of treatment, such as ANH. Where members of the team have a conscientious objection to the withdrawal of life-prolonging treatment they should, wherever possible, be permitted to hand over their role in the care of such patients to colleagues. Where, however, an individual does not disagree in principle with withdrawing or withholding life-prolonging treatment but considers the action to be unjustified in a particular case and can produce reasonable arguments to that effect, further discussion will be required to attempt to resolve this conflict, possibly by seeking a further medical opinion or independent review.

17. Resource management

17.1. Health professionals have an ethical duty to make the best use of available resources. This inevitably means that some patients, whose lives might be prolonged, may not receive all possible life-prolonging treatment. Decisions must represent an appropriate balance between the clinical and resource needs of different patients. As with all decisions doctors must be able to justify their actions and show that decisions were made fairly and not on the basis of unjustifiable discrimination.

Increasing levels of technology not only present ethical dilemmas about assessing when treatment ceases to benefit the patient but also raise the issue of withholding or withdrawing potentially beneficial treatment on grounds of cost. Where funds are limited, individual hospitals, doctors and patients are competing for resources. Particular difficulties could arise if, for example, patients or their families request life-prolonging treatment to be continued for as long as technically possible, even though there is no hope of recovery. Complying with such requests could be at the expense of other patients who have a reasonable chance of recovery if treatment is provided. Taking account of all relevant factors, the decision about whether to offer treatment is ultimately made by the clinician (medical or nursing) in charge of the patient's care with advice from the rest of the health care team. This is part of their role as 'gatekeepers' to treatment, which obliges health professionals to balance the clinical and resource needs of different patients. This includes assessing the likelihood of prolonging life leading to a significant recovery for one patient against the likelihood of merely delaying death for a short period of time or prolonging the dying process for another.

Although it is unlikely that the courts would expect all possible treatment that could prolong life to be given, irrespective of costs or the impact on other patients, no clear guidance has been provided on this specific point. In Burke (see Section 5), the duty of care owed to patients with capacity was said to include taking 'reasonable' steps to prolong the patient's life; what is 'reasonable' is a matter for judgement but it can be assumed that it will involve taking account of the resource implications of such decisions. The duty of care owed to patients who lack capacity is to act in their best interests but competing demands on limited resources and the concomitant but competing best interests of other patients are factors that need to be taken into consideration. It is improbable that the courts will turn the guarantee of the right to life in the Human Rights Act (see Section 18) into a positive obligation to supply all life-prolonging treatments to all patients regardless of the resources available [36].

Until clear advice is provided from the courts about the extent of the doctor's duty to prolong life and the legitimate role of resource management issues in such decisions, a decision to withhold or withdraw life-prolonging treatment on resource grounds could be open to legal challenge and must be well supported by clinical evidence, second opinions and by reference to national or local guidelines. Such decisions should be discussed, in advance, with senior clinical and managerial colleagues. Particular care needs to be taken to ensure that all decisions have been carefully considered and are not made on the basis of unjustifiable discrimination.

Part 3 **Legal and ethical considerations that apply to all decisions to withhold or withdraw treatment**

There are some important legal and ethical considerations that are common to all decisions to withhold or withdraw life-prolonging treatment throughout the UK. These issues are discussed in this section which sets the framework within which individual decisions must be made.

18. Human Rights Act 1998

18.1. The Human Rights Act 1998 came fully into force throughout the UK in October 2000. As a result, all public authorities are required to act in accordance with the rights set out in the Human Rights Act, and all statutes have to be interpreted so far as possible to be in accordance with those rights.

When the Act first came into force there was some uncertainty about whether all doctors are considered to be 'public authorities', who are bound by the terms of the Human Rights Act, by virtue of the nature of the service they provide. It now appears that doctors who are providing a wholly private service (and not providing services on behalf of the NHS) are not bound by its terms [37]. Given that the Act reflects good medical practice, however, we believe that all health professionals and health teams, howsoever constituted, should practise as though they are bound by the terms of the Human Rights Act.

The rights that are most relevant to decisions to withhold or withdraw life-prolonging treatment are:

Article 2 – the right to life

Article 3 – the right not to be tortured or subjected to inhuman or degrading treatment

Article 5 – the right to security of the person

Article 8 – the right to respect for privacy and family life

Article 9 – the right to freedom of thought, conscience and religion

Article 10 – the right to freedom of expression including the right to receive and impart information

Article 14 – the right not to be discriminated against in the enjoyment of these various rights.

Under the Human Rights Act, public authorities are bound in relation to their omissions as well as their actions [38].

18.2. The basic principles that underpin the Human Rights Act – most significantly respect for human dignity and respect for legality – are the same ideas that underpin much of the ethical and legal framework for withholding and withdrawing life-prolonging treatment.

In the second edition of this guidance we speculated that the impact of human rights legislation would be less dramatic in this field than in other areas of law. This was because the requirements of the Human Rights Act reflect, very closely, existing good medical practice. This prediction has been largely realised in cases that have tested the human rights' compliance of decisions to withhold or withdraw treatment. The main difference between recent judgments and those prior to the Human Rights Act has been in the language used and the more explicit consideration of human rights arguments, rather than differences in the outcome of such analysis. Nevertheless, this difference is an important one and health professionals need to be aware of the Human Rights Act and ensure that they are able to demonstrate compliance with it in any particular case.

18.3.   Health professionals need to be mindful of the ways in which the basic rights set out in the Human Rights Act might impinge on their decision making. Frequently different rights conflict and health professionals must be able to demonstrate that they have balanced the duties and obligations imposed by those rights and have reached a reasonable and proportionate decision.

This section sets out aspects of decisions to withhold or withdraw life-prolonging treatment that are likely to engage the basic rights set out in the Human Rights Act. Although this guidance closely reflects what is already established good practice, it is important that doctors are aware of the Human Rights Act, are familiar with its language and are able to demonstrate that their decisions are consistent with its terms.

Article 2 – the right to life
Under the Human Rights Act '[E]veryone's right to life shall be protected by law' (Article 2(1)). This is a positive obligation to preserve life as well as a negative order not to kill, but the positive obligation is not one that should be pushed too far. The Article 2(1) guarantee does not involve an absolute obligation indefinitely to prolong life at all costs and without regard to the consequences for the patient of such a prolongation.

Until 2004, the European Court had avoided making a decision as to whether 'everyone' whose life is protected extended to the unborn child. It addressed this issue in the case of Vo v. France in which the European Court of Human Rights clearly stated that the Article 2 right to life does not extend to an unborn fetus, but rather the protection to be afforded to the fetus is a matter to be decided by individual states [39]. This confirmed the Human Rights Act compliance of existing case law that a pregnant woman with capacity is entitled to refuse any treatment even if that refusal would result in the death of her fetus (see Section 25.6).

Article 3 – the right to be free from inhuman and degrading treatment

In addition to the Human Rights Act's guarantee of protection for life it also declares that '[N]o one shall be subjected to torture or to inhuman or degrading treatment or punishment' (Article 3). Life should not be artificially preserved where the treatment to secure this leaves a patient in what might be judged as 'an inhuman or degrading state'. Article 3 may, for example, be engaged where parents or relatives insist on providing all possible treatment to keep a patient alive. Consideration should be given to whether acceding to such requests would involve the possibility of subjecting the patient to inhuman or degrading treatment, in contravention of Article 3. Article 3 could also be engaged if the withdrawal of treatment leaves patients in a situation that amounts to inhuman or degrading treatment.

Doctors must balance their duty to protect life with their obligation not to subject the patient to inhuman or degrading treatment. Guidance from the courts about how to interpret Article 3 is, however, unclear and in fact two different views have emerged. When considering the withdrawal of artificial nutrition and hydration from two patients in persistent vegetative state, Lady Justice Butler-Sloss said:

> 'I am, moreover, satisfied that Article 3 requires the victim to be aware of the inhuman and degrading treatment which he or she is experiencing or at least to be in a state of physical or mental suffering. An insensate patient suffering from permanent vegetative state has no feelings and no comprehension of the treatment accorded to him or her. Article 3 does not in my judgement apply to these cases.' [40]

This interpretation was, however, subsequently rejected by Mr Justice Munby in the case of Burke v. GMC, where he said:

> '... however unconscious or unaware of ill-treatment a particular incompetent adult or a baby may be, treatment which has the effect on those who witness it of degrading the individual may come within

> Article 3. Otherwise . . . *the Convention's emphasis on the protection of the vulnerable may be circumvented.*' [41]

Although Mr Munby's overall decision in the case was subsequently over-turned by the Court of Appeal and no further comment was made on this aspect of the judgment, many legal commentators accept this latter interpre-tation of Article 3 as being more in keeping with the aims of human rights legislation. Health care teams would be well advised to err on the side of caution and to take account of Mr Munby's interpretation of Article 3 when making treatment and non-treatment decisions.

The courts have made clear that Article 3 provides the right to 'dignity in death'. This was established in a case heard shortly before the implementation of the Human Rights Act, in which a health care team sought approval to withhold artificial ventilation from a baby boy despite the objection of his parents [42]. Referring back to previous cases in which non-treatment had been found to be in the best interests of the child, the High Court held that it would be lawful for artificial ventilation to be withheld if, in the opinion of the treating paediatrician, that was clinically appropriate. The judge went on to say that withholding this treatment did not conflict with the Human Rights Act. The judge was of the view that there could be no infringement of the right to life (Article 2) because withholding artificial ventilation was in the baby's best interests, and the right to be free from inhuman or degrading treatment (Article 3) included a right to 'dignity in death'.

Article 5 – the right to security of the person
Where a patient has capacity and refuses treatment, that person's right to security of the person in Article 5 and the right to respect for privacy in Article 8 override any duty on the doctor to preserve life (under Article 2). This also extends to respecting a valid advance refusal of treatment made by an adult patient with capacity.

Article 8 – the right to private and family life
In addition to the right of patients with capacity to refuse treatment, Article 8 also ensures the right to confidentiality. So, where a patient with capacity has expressed a specific wish that his or her condition should not be discussed with relatives or friends, this should be respected even when capacity is lost. Where the patient has not expressed such a wish, it is likely that Article 8 gives those close to patients the right to be consulted about treatment decisions. (This point is also reinforced in England and Wales by the Mental Capacity Act (see Section 27) and in Scotland by the Adults with Incapacity (Scotland) Act (see Section 31).) This right may also extend to parents who do not have parental

responsibility even though they lack the legal authority to give consent on behalf of children. This right to be consulted, however, does not mean that their views are determinative and their wishes need to be balanced against the doctor's obligations under Articles 2 and 3.

Article 9 – the right to freedom of thought, conscience and religion

The right of doctors to claim a conscientious objection to certain forms of medical treatment is reinforced by the right to freedom of conscience and religion which is to be found in Article 9. This is, however, subject to restriction where 'necessary in a democratic society' for, among other reasons, 'the protection of health' and the 'protection of . . . the rights and freedoms of others'.

Some people's views about the withdrawal or withholding of treatment are based on strongly held religious convictions and their right to have these views respected is also guaranteed by Article 9. Where the decision is being made on behalf of another person such as parents deciding for a child, however, this might be overridden by the obligations of the health care team under Article 2 or Article 3 as was the case in Re C (see Section 47.7).

Article 10 – the right to receive and impart information

In addition to being good medical practice, and important for ensuring the validity of consent, the provision of accurate information is also a requirement of the Human Rights Act. Patients, and parents of children who lack capacity, have a right under Article 10 to receive information that is relevant to their condition in a way they can understand, in order to help them to make informed decisions.

Article 14 – the right to be free from discrimination in the enjoyment of these rights

Article 14 is not a stand-alone right but relates to discrimination in the enjoyment of one of the other rights. So, for example, if a decision to withhold life-prolonging medical treatment is made on the basis of unjustifiable discrimination, this would represent a breach of that individual's enjoyment of their Article 2 right to life and so would potentially breach Article 14 and Article 2. It is, of course, entirely appropriate that individuals are treated differently based on their individual circumstances although this could be described as discrimination. Discrimination only engages Article 14 where it involves unjustified differences in the treatment of individuals in comparable situations – what is often referred to as 'unjustifiable discrimination'. Examples of unjustifiable discrimination would include differences based solely on factors such as age, gender, race, religion, sexuality or disability.

Summary – Human Rights Act

- *All health professionals should act as though they are bound by the Human Rights Act*
- *The Human Rights Act very closely reflects good ethical practice*
- *Doctors must be familiar with the terms of the Act and the language of rights in order to be able to demonstrate that their decisions are compliant with the legislation*
- *Where rights conflict, health professionals must be able to demonstrate that they have balanced the conflicting rights and reached a reasonable and proportionate decision*

---

19. Fairness and non-discrimination

19.1. In addition to the legal duty to avoid discriminating unjustifiably against patients, there is also a professional and ethical duty to ensure that decisions to withhold or withdraw treatment are made on the basis of a proper assessment of the relevant factors in each individual case. Decisions must not be made on the basis of assumptions based solely on factors such as the patient's age or disability.

All patients are entitled to a fair and unprejudiced assessment of their individual situation. The General Medical Council's guidance, which is binding on doctors, states very clearly that:

> *'Doctors have a duty to give priority to patients on the basis of clinical need, while seeking to make the best use of resources using up to date evidence about the clinical efficacy of treatments. Doctors must not allow their views about, for example, a patient's age, disability, race, colour, culture, beliefs, sexuality, gender, lifestyle, social or economic status to prejudice the choices of treatment offered or the general standard of care provided.'* [43]

It is undoubtedly the case that decisions to withhold or withdraw life-prolonging treatment are more common among older patients. This is not because of their age per se, but because older patients are more likely to have multiple morbidity and, because of their clinical condition, may be unable to withstand the risks associated with certain forms of treatment (such as general anaesthetic). While the reasons for withholding or withdrawing treatment are clear to the clinical team involved in making the decision, there is a risk that they could appear to reflect unjustifiable discrimination. It is therefore essential that the reasons for reaching a decision not to provide life-prolonging treatment are clearly articulated, recorded in the notes and explained to patients who have capacity or those close to, or representing, patients in whom capacity is lacking.

The same applies to patients who have disabilities, where decisions are made on the basis of the clinical factors in each case and not simply on the basis of the disability. Medical staff have in the past been criticised by the courts for the basis of their decisions. In the case of NHS Trust v. S, Lady Justice Butler-Sloss said:

> 'The Hospital Trust has, very properly, made it clear that it has always recognised the right of S to be treated as fairly as any other patient without his disabilities. ... But the approach of the medical and nursing team, both in the paediatric unit and in the adult unit, has been coloured by their real difficulties in the lack of verbal communication with S and their vivid recollections of how difficult he was to manage in the hospital after he was admitted for emergency lifesaving treatment in May 2000. I have the feeling that those difficulties may have had a disproportionate effect upon their approach to future treatment for S.' [44]

NHS Trust v. S

S was 18 years old and had been born with a genetic condition, velo-cardiac-facial syndrome. His problems included severe developmental delay, bilateral renal dysplasia, autism, epilepsy and moderate immunodeficiency. Despite these problems he lived at home with his family, was able to look after himself to some extent, attended a special school and was able to take part in school activities. In May 2000 he was admitted to hospital with acute renal failure and had been on haemodialysis ever since. In this time, the hospital staff had found S difficult to manage, he was sometimes aggressive and violent towards his mother and nursing staff, he had pulled out tubes and lines and on occasions had to be physically restrained. S had limited understanding of his medical condition, became very distressed by changes to his routine, had very limited communication skills and lacked the capacity to make decisions about his future treatment. The hospital originally sought a declaration that in the event that haemodialysis could no longer be provided, neither peritoneal dialysis nor a kidney transplant would be in S's best interests and only palliative care should be provided.

As the case progressed some agreement was reached and the remaining areas of disagreement to be considered by the court were whether a kidney transplant would ever be suitable for S and whether haemodialysis by an AV fistula would be appropriate. A principal concern of the medical team in relation to transplantation was S's ability to understand and cope with major surgery and the necessary long-term follow-up treatment. Others who gave evidence, some of whom knew S well and had experience of patients with similar disabilities, felt that he could understand and cope with such an operation if he was given time and assistance.

Butler-Sloss LJ held that haemodialysis should be continued for as long as possible. The possibility of an AV fistula should not be excluded and, subject to the medical evidence at the time, kidney transplantation should not be ruled out. The judge criticised the hospital staff for giving too much weight to the difficulties they had encountered with S's behaviour in the past.

NHS Trust v. (1) S (2) DG (3) SG [45]

19.2.   When assessing treatment options decision makers must not be unduly influenced by any of their own pre-existing negative views about living with a particular condition or disability.

The Disability Rights Commission (DRC) intervened in the case of Mr Burke (see Section 5) saying 'some decisions by medical professionals on whether disabled people should live or die are based on a backdrop of negative images and poorly informed assumptions of intolerable suffering and unacceptable dependence on others; and a fear that "quality of life" decisions are sometimes based on the assumption that a particular disability makes life not worth living'. [46] To illustrate their case the DRC referred to the case of a woman who has spinal muscular atrophy and, although severely disabled, is living a fulfilling and productive life. In 2003 she was struck down with pneumonia and the DRC reported that two consultants were minded to conclude that her life was so parlous that if she needed artificial respiration to stay alive she would not wish to receive it. The consultants were persuaded to the contrary after discussion with her husband who showed them a photograph of her taking her degree.

Whether or not the criticisms levelled against doctors are justified, the DRC raises an important point for everyone making such decisions to bear in mind. What is important is not the decision maker's view of the disability or what he or she would want in the same situation but an objective assessment of what is in the best interests of the particular patient taking account of all relevant factors.

19.3.   When assessing treatment options, the benefits, risks and burdens of treatment must be assessed in each individual case.

Evaluation must be undertaken on a case-by-case basis rather than assuming that the same treatment decisions will be appropriate for all patients with a particular condition or of a particular age. This judgement must take account of all relevant medical, ethical and legal considerations and best established practice in that area. Decision making should be transparent and able to withstand close scrutiny.

Summary – Fairness and non-discrimination

- *All patients are entitled to a fair and unprejudiced assessment of their individual situation*
- *Doctors must not allow their views of the patient's age, disability, race, sexuality or lifestyle to prejudice the choice of treatments offered*
- *The reasons for withholding or withdrawing treatment should be clearly articulated, recorded and explained to avoid misunderstanding and the perception of unjustifiable discrimination*
- *Health professionals must not be unduly influenced by their own pre-existing negative views about living with a particular condition or disability*

---

20. Communication

20.1. Good communication is an essential part of decision making.

Good communication is a vitally important aspect of decisions to withhold or withdraw life-prolonging treatment. Experience shows that conflict and disagreement are frequently the result of poor communication and inadequate provision of accurate information. Discussion should always include patients and, with due regard to confidentiality (see Section 21), those close to, or representing, patients who lack capacity to make or communicate a decision. Information should be provided sensitively and in a way that can be easily understood by those who do not have medical training or a detailed knowledge of the condition. Some patients may need additional help and support to understand and assess the information provided, such as the young, the elderly, those with disabilities that affect their level of comprehension and those for whom English is not their first language. Every effort should be made to meet the specific information needs of each patient, using interpreters or advocates as appropriate. Information should be made available in different formats to accommodate the needs of those with a range of impairments, including easy read and graphic facilitation for people with learning difficulties, and Braille, large print and audio for people with visual impairments.

Communication involves listening as well as providing information and health professionals should encourage those consulted to ask questions and to actively contribute to the decision-making process. Patients should be encouraged to be involved in decision making to the extent to which they feel comfortable. Where the patient is a child, or an adult who lacks capacity, parents, others close to the patient, welfare attorneys, deputies or advocates should be consulted. Those consulted must be made aware of their role in relation to the decision and there should be no ambiguity about who has the final responsibility for making treatment decisions.

20.2. An explanation should be given to patients and those close to them about why treatment is given and why, in some circumstances, a decision to withhold or withdraw further life-prolonging treatment may need to be considered.

When treatment fails or ceases to provide a net benefit to the patient, the primary justification for continuing to provide it no longer exists. Wherever possible any decision should involve sensitive and detailed discussion with the patient. Where the patient lacks capacity and, following appropriate consultation with those close to, or representing, the patient, a decision has been made to withhold or withdraw a particular treatment, the reasons for this should be carefully explained so that it is not interpreted as 'giving up' on or abandoning the patient. To minimise the perception that the patient is being abandoned, attention should be given to explaining the care that is available including, for example, palliative care.

It is important that all those involved in the decision understand why the decision has been made, on what grounds and with what implications. Doctors have an obligation not only to ensure that reliable data are used to make the decision but also to ensure that those data can be accessed by everyone closely involved in the decision.

Summary – Communication

- *Good communication is an essential part of decision making*
- *Health professionals should encourage those consulted to ask questions and to actively contribute to the decision-making process*
- *Information should be provided sensitively and in a way that is easily understood by those without medical training*

---

21. Confidentiality

21.1. Doctors have a duty of confidentiality to all of their patients irrespective of age or disability.

21.2. Information about patients with capacity should not be shared with other family members without their consent.

Where patients have capacity it is for them to decide with whom they share information about their illness, prognosis and treatment. It is not unusual for relatives of elderly, young or very sick patients to request that information is given to them alone to avoid distressing the patient. It is important to explain that the primary duty of the health care team is to the patient and if he or she has capacity, information may not be shared with other family members without the patient's consent.

21.3. Where patients lack capacity it is usually reasonable to assume that they would want people close to them to be given information about their illness, prognosis and treatment unless there is evidence to the contrary.

Where a patient is seriously ill and lacks capacity it would be unreasonable to always refuse to provide any information to those close to the patient on the basis that the individual had not given explicit consent. This does not, however, mean that all information should be routinely shared and where the information is sensitive, a judgement will be needed about how much information the patient is likely to want passed on to whom. Where there is evidence that the patient did not want information shared, this must be respected.

Those close to, or representing, patients who lack capacity have an important part to play in decision making, whether they have a formal role as a proxy decision maker, welfare attorney or advocate, or more informally in terms of helping the health care team to assess the patient's best interests. It is not possible to carry out this role without some information being provided about the medical condition of the patient.

Summary – Confidentiality

- *Doctors have a duty of confidentiality to all of their patients irrespective of age or disability*
- *Where patients have capacity information should not be shared with their relatives without the patient's consent*
- *Where patients lack capacity information may be shared with those close to or representing them unless there is evidence that this would be contrary to the patient's wishes*

22. Legal review

22.1. In the vast majority of cases agreement is reached about the best way to proceed but, where disagreement arises, steps should be taken to address the issue without delay. Further information, discussion and seeking a second opinion can resolve some difficulties but where these mechanisms fail legal advice should be sought.

Although media reporting of high-profile legal cases may appear daunting to health professionals, patients and their families, many disagreements can be resolved without the need for a full court hearing. Sometimes lawyers are able to give advice about how to proceed or a judge may make a decision without a full hearing, for example, in a medical emergency where an urgent decision is needed in the middle of the night. It is important to remember that the law can provide a protective role for both patients and the health care team who treat them and where there is disagreement that cannot be resolved, legal advice should be sought without delay in order that the matter may be resolved. Health professionals should not be deterred from seeking a legal ruling because of the risk of appearing confrontational; legal review can be beneficial for all parties. It is also important to remember that doctors have been criticised in the past for failing to seek advice from the courts where there was disagreement about the best course of action (see Section 47.8). Where a judge is asked to make a declaration, it is important that all parties are kept informed of developments and are given information about how their views can be represented.

22.2. In reaching a judgement about best interests, the courts are increasingly using a 'balance sheet' approach and this can be a useful exercise for health professionals to consider in the event of disagreement.

The Court of Appeal, in cases such as that of Charlotte Wyatt (see Section 48.1), has suggested that the best and safest way of reliably weighing up all of the factors in order to assess best interests is to draw up a list on which are specifically identified on one side the benefits or advantages and on the other side the burdens or disadvantages of continuing or discontinuing the treatment [47]. In the case of baby MB (see Section 47.7) the judge asked each of the parties in the case to compile and submit such a list. The exercise is not a numerical one; as Mr Justice Holman said in that case, the difficulty and real dispute is how much weight to attach to particular items. The list Holman LJ quotes has 6 benefits to continuing treatment (and therefore staying alive) and 27 burdens or harms but the weight he attached to those advantages swung the balance in favour of continuing treatment [48]. This methodology, increasingly used by the courts, can be a helpful way of ensuring that all of the relevant factors are considered.

22.3. Where professional guidance is available which represents the views of a responsible body of medical opinion, this may be used by doctors and the courts to determine the acceptability of a particular practice.

In many legal cases concerning treatment, judges rely on professional medical guidance or codes of practice in reaching decisions. Professional guidance, which represents the views of a responsible body of medical opinion, can provide important information and advice about good practice and may be adopted by the courts in a particular case although it does not, in itself, have legal standing. Whilst professional guidance cannot be followed blindly, if it has a logical basis and is factually correct, a doctor acting in accordance with the guidance in a particular case is likely to be seen to have acted reasonably. The acceptability of a particular treatment (judged by the standard of what most doctors would find reasonable – the 'Bolam test') is not, however, the same as whether the treatment is in a patient's best interests (see Sections 9 and 40).

Existing resources should also be utilised where additional advice is needed. General advice may be provided in individual cases by professional bodies, such as the BMA and the relevant Royal Colleges, defence bodies, Trust solicitors, the Office of the Official Solicitor (in England, Wales and Northern Ireland) and the Mental Welfare Commission or NHS Central Legal Office (in Scotland) where the patient lacks capacity and the Children and Family Court Advisory and Support Service (CAFCASS) in England and Wales, where the patient is a child.

Part 4 **Medical considerations that apply to all decisions to withhold or withdraw treatment**

23. Medical assessment

23.1. For all patients, treatment decisions, including those to withhold or withdraw life-prolonging treatment, must be based on reliable clinical evidence.

Factual information should be collected about the patient's condition, diagnosis and prognosis including the stability of the patient's condition over a period of time and the underlying pathology. Wherever possible, the assessment of the patient's condition should be evidence based and carried out according to best practice.

It is vital that research findings on treatment outcomes are made widely available and that, through continuing professional education, doctors ensure that they keep up to date with new developments. Doctors also have obligations to undergo a process of revalidation of their skills both for their own protection and that of their patients.

23.2. Where relevant locally or nationally agreed guidelines exist for the diagnosis and management of the condition, these should be consulted as part of the clinical assessment. Additional advice should be sought where necessary.

There is currently a limited number of conditions for which guidelines are available but there is a need for more to be developed. Where guidelines are not available and there is reasonable doubt about the diagnosis or prognosis or where the health care team has limited experience of the condition, particularly with comparatively rare disorders, advice should be sought from another senior clinician with experience of the condition before making decisions about withdrawing or withholding life-prolonging treatment. Where, for example, assessments are required about the extent of brain damage and the likelihood of any degree of recovery, advice will usually be required from a clinician with expertise in the long-term consequences and management of brain injury.

In case of challenge or disagreement, health professionals must be able to demonstrate a reasonable justification for their decisions including those which deviate from established guidance. Detailed notes should be kept of any guidelines consulted or additional opinions sought.

23.3. Despite being evidence based, some aspects of medical treatment will always remain uncertain. Although death is a certainty for everyone, diagnosis and prognosis are based on probability and past evidence rather than absolute certainty.

Much fear is engendered by reports of mistaken diagnosis or a belief that had treatment been provided, the patient might have recovered to a level that would have been acceptable to that individual. One of the difficulties for health professionals is that it is often not possible to predict with certainty how any individual will respond to a particular treatment or, in the final stages of an illness, how long the dying process will take. Health professionals have an ethical and professional obligation to keep their skills up to date and to keep abreast of new developments in their specialty and to base their decisions on a reasonable assessment of the facts available. There will, however, always remain some areas of uncertainty and empirical judgements are necessarily based on probabilities rather than certainties. Wider consultation, including a second opinion, should be sought where the treating doctor has doubt about the proposed decision.

Part of the discussion between the health care team and patients with capacity or those close to or representing patients who lack capacity should include frank but sensitive discussion about the fact that medicine is not a precise science and it is often impossible to predict with certainty how any particular person will respond to treatment or how the disease will progress.

23.4. Although ultimately the responsibility for deciding what treatment to offer rests with the clinician in charge of the patient's care, it is important, where non-emergency decisions are made, that account is taken of the views of other health professionals involved in the patient's care.

The importance of team working in providing health care is widely recognised and is particularly important when making complex decisions about whether to withhold or withdraw life-prolonging treatment. Seeking agreement within the team about the most appropriate course of action can help to reduce the possibility of subjectivity or bias in cases of uncertainty. All health professionals involved with caring for the patient have an important contribution to make to the assessment; nurses often have a particular insight into the patient's wishes and may have spent considerable time with the patient and the patient's relatives. Many nurses have reported concern about what they perceive as 'moral distancing' on the part of some doctors. They consider that those who make the decision generally delegate its implementation to nurses, who can feel unhappy if they have not been able to contribute to that decision. Depending upon the type of treatment under consideration, it may be appropriate to involve a dietician, speech therapist, psychologist, physiotherapist and other members of the team who have been involved in the patient's care. Where patients lack capacity, their general practitioner might be able to provide valuable information about the patients' wishes or values. General practice notes may, for example, include discussions with the patient about future treatment, particularly if the patient was aware that he or she was suffering from a progressive illness in the period before decision-making capacity, or the ability to communicate, was lost.

23.5. Where the patient has an existing condition which means that the progression of the disorder is known or it is recognised that cardiac arrest is likely, consideration should be given in advance to formulating a management plan to anticipate such events. Such plans should be discussed with patients who have capacity and with those close to or representing patients who lack capacity including sensitively informing them when a decision is made not to resuscitate because the patient would not survive the resuscitation attempt. Any such decisions, and the reasons for them, should be recorded in the medical notes.

Advance planning for anticipated medical events or the progression of the disorder allows more time for discussion with the patient (or, where the patient lacks capacity, with those close to or representing the patient) and for discussion and reflection within the health care team. This avoids the need to make decisions abruptly. One common example of advance planning concerns decisions relating to cardiopulmonary resuscitation, which is the subject of separate guidance from the BMA [49].

Summary – Medical assessment

- *Treatment decisions must be based on reliable clinical evidence*
- *Where there is doubt about the diagnosis or prognosis, advice should be sought from another senior clinician with relevant specialist experience*
- *Doctors should be honest with patients, their relatives or advocates about the uncertainty that is inherent in medical practice*
- *Wherever possible advance care plans should be discussed and agreed*

---

24. Medical decision making

24.1. All treatment decisions for patients at the end of life should be made in the context of the provision of good quality palliative care.

24.2. In emergency situations where there is doubt about the appropriateness of treatment and no prior decision has been made, there should be a presumption in favour of providing life-prolonging treatment even though this may be withdrawn at a later stage when more information is available.

Where a patient presents with a sudden or unexpected medical event, there is likely to be initial uncertainty about the diagnosis, the likely effectiveness of treatment and the long-term prognosis. In these cases, the initial efforts should be focused on stabilising the patient, so that a proper assessment of the condition may be undertaken, the likelihood and extent of any expected improvement can be assessed and the patient's wishes can be ascertained. In the immediate aftermath of an accident, injury, stroke or onset of an unexpected condition, for example, the initial efforts are aimed at stabilising the patient's condition to allow time for a proper assessment. Time is an important factor in relation to recovery rates for many medical conditions, and questions about the continuation or initiation of treatment are more likely to arise when patients fail to demonstrate any improvement over a prolonged period.

24.3. Where treatment is able to restore or maintain the patient to a level of health that he or she would find acceptable, then active treatment is clearly appropriate.

24.4. Where treatment is unable to achieve any clinical benefit to the patient, for example because it is unable to achieve its physiological aim, the health care team should not offer it.

24.5. Where treatment is unable to restore or maintain the patient to a level of health that he or she would find acceptable, active treatment may not be appropriate.

Where the decision to withhold or withdraw treatment is based on the lack of any clinical benefit then this is clearly a matter for the health care team. Patients with capacity and those close to or representing patients who lack capacity should be sensitively informed of the decision not to provide or to continue the treatment and the reasons for it. They may ask for a second opinion or further discussion but they cannot insist that clinically inappropriate treatment is provided.

Where the decision to withhold treatment is made principally on 'quality of life' considerations (see Section 6) or on the basis of the level of recovery that would be acceptable to the patient, this is not just a matter for health professionals. Where patients have capacity they are the best judges of whether the quality of life that could be achieved is acceptable to them. Where the patient lacks capacity, the level of recovery that would be acceptable to the patient must be the subject of discussion and agreement between the health care team and those close to or representing the patient where this is possible within the time available. In practice, however, the distinction between clinical and overall benefit is not always clear-cut. In some cases, for example, there may be a small chance of improvement in the patient's condition but also the risk of harm to the patient, or the treatment may prolong the patient's life for a short period but with severe side-effects. The balance between clinical and other considerations that need to be considered vary in each case and doctors need to consider the individual circumstances to determine who has responsibility for making the decision. Where there is any doubt, or where there is an element of these broader best interests considerations to the decision, patients themselves, or those close to or representing patients lacking capacity, should be involved with making the decision.

24.6. Where there is reasonable doubt about its potential for benefit, treatment should be provided for a trial period with a subsequent pre-arranged review. If, following the review, it is decided that the treatment has failed or ceased to be of benefit to the patient, consideration should be given to its withdrawal.

Where insufficient information is available about the severity of the condition or the likelihood of recovery at the time a decision is needed, treatment should be provided although this may be for a trial period with a pre-arranged review. With stroke patients, for example, where the outcome is uncertain, all appropriate treatment, including artificial nutrition and hydration, should usually be provided in order to stabilise the patient to give time for proper assessment. The treatment may, however, be withdrawn following a review after a pre-determined period, if it is agreed that the patient's condition is so severe that the burdens of providing the treatment outweigh the benefits. A decision should be made, in advance, about when the review will take place and the factors that will be taken into account in deciding whether to continue to provide treatment after the review.

Information about such 'trials of treatment' should be sensitively shared with patients or (with due regard to confidentiality – see Section 21) with those close to or representing patients lacking capacity.

24.7. Treatment should never be withheld merely on the grounds that it is easier to withhold treatment than to withdraw treatment which has been initiated.

It is unacceptable to withhold any treatment, including artificial nutrition and hydration, on the grounds that it is considered easier (for example, for the family to accept) to withhold the treatment than to withdraw that which has already been started. Similarly, a non-beneficial treatment should not be provided for the sake of the family.

24.8. Except where the patient's imminent death is inevitable or a competent patient has refused all treatment, a decision to withhold or withdraw *all* treatment is likely to be inappropriate and potentially unlawful. Assessments should be based on whether each potentially available treatment would benefit the patient, taking account of the residual effect of any remaining medication or treatment on the patient.

An important part of the assessment includes consideration of the effect of continuing to provide some treatment in isolation from the medical procedure being withdrawn. Where ventilatory support is to be withdrawn, for example, consideration must be given to the continuing residual effect of any medication which has been provided which has the effect of suppressing the patient's ability to breathe unaided. Failure to do so could be interpreted, in law, as action taken with the purpose, objective or intention of ending the patient's life.

24.9. Where the patient's imminent death is inevitable, active treatment (including artificial nutrition or hydration) may no longer provide benefit to the patient and may be withheld or withdrawn.

Once an individual's condition has reached the stage where death is imminent, such as in the final stages of a terminal illness, the focus of care changes from attempting to prolong life to keeping the patient as comfortable as possible until death occurs. In these final stages, active treatment and the provision of artificial nutrition and/or hydration may become unnecessarily intrusive and merely prolong the dying process rather than offering a benefit to the patient. Basic care and palliation of distressing symptoms should, however, always be provided (including the offer of oral nutrition and hydration). Efforts should be made to make the patient as comfortable as possible. The basis on which the decision to withdraw or withhold treatment was made, and subsequent action, should be recorded in the medical notes.

24.10. All treatment decisions should be reviewed on a regular basis both before and after implementation.

Regular review should be undertaken by the clinician in charge of the patient's care in consultation with the rest of the health care team to take account of any changing circumstances before or after implementation of the decision. Decisions should also be subject to audit to ensure that appropriate procedures were followed and that the decisions were properly documented.

Summary – Medical decision making

- *All treatment decisions at the end of life should be made in the context of the provision of good quality palliative care*
- *In emergency situations where there is doubt about benefit, there is a presumption in favour of providing life-prolonging treatment although it may later be withdrawn*
- *Treatment should never be withheld simply because it is easier to withhold it than to withdraw treatment that has been initiated*
- *Except where the patient's imminent death is inevitable or a competent patient has refused all treatment, a decision to withdraw all treatment is likely to be unacceptable and potentially unlawful*

Part 5 **Decision making by adults with capacity**

In many ways decisions involving adults with capacity are the most straight-forward since there is opportunity for discussion with patients about what risks, burdens and side-effects they are prepared to tolerate and what level of recovery they would find acceptable. The most important factors are communication and information – ensuring that patients have all the necessary information and support to make informed decisions.

25. The law

25.1. In law, young people have the same rights as adults to give or withhold consent to treatment from the age of 18 in England, Wales and Northern Ireland and the age of 16 in Scotland. For information about decision making by those under these ages, see Part 7.

25.2. There is a legal presumption that adults have the capacity to make decisions unless the contrary is proven.

Patients are entitled to make decisions that conflict with the views of the health care team. The fact that an individual has made a decision which appears to others to be irrational or unjustified should not necessarily be taken as evidence that the individual lacks the mental capacity to make that decision. If, however, the decision is clearly contrary to previously expressed wishes or is based on a misperception of reality such as, for example, believing that the blood is poisoned because it is red [50], this may be indicative of a lack of the requisite capacity and further investigation will be required. Health professionals should try to ensure that patients understand the likely consequences of their decisions and are not acting under any misapprehension. More information about assessing and maximising capacity, where there is doubt, is given in Section 38.

25.3. Although patients' wishes should always be discussed with them, the fact that a patient has requested a particular treatment does not mean that it must always be provided.

Doctors are not obliged to offer treatment that is clinically inappropriate and nor are they required to provide all possible treatment to keep patients alive. The extent of the health care team's duty of care is discussed in Section 5.

25.4. Provided it is able to achieve its physiological aim, artificial nutrition and/or hydration should never be withdrawn or withheld from a patient with capacity who has expressed a wish to remain alive. The provision of artificial nutrition and hydration (ANH) in these circumstances will always provide a benefit for the patient.

In the case of Burke v. GMC (see Section 5) the Court of Appeal stated that where a patient with capacity requests ANH this must, in almost all circumstances, be provided. It is difficult to know how far the principles established in that case can be extrapolated to other life-prolonging treatments and other circumstances. If a patient with capacity requests any life-prolonging treatment (such as artificial ventilation) that is able to achieve its physiological aim, then the expectation would be that the treatment would be provided. The courts have not, however, specifically addressed the resource issues raised by the duty to prolong life where that is the patient's wish but for doctors involved with providing care, these will be serious considerations (see Section 17).

Advance requests for life-prolonging treatment, including artificial nutrition or hydration, should be taken into consideration in assessing best interests but are not necessarily determinative.

25.5. A voluntary refusal of life-prolonging treatment by an adult with capacity must be respected. Legally, to provide treatment for an adult with capacity without his or her consent, or in the face of a valid refusal, would constitute battery or assault and could result in legal action being taken against the doctor. It may also involve a breach of the patient's human rights.

It is well established in law and ethics that adults with capacity have the right to refuse any medical treatment, even if that refusal results in their death. Patients are not obliged to justify their decisions but the health team usually wish to discuss the refusal with them in order to ensure that they have based their decisions on accurate information and to correct any misunderstandings. Where the health team considers that the treatment would provide a net benefit, that assessment should be sympathetically explained to the patient but patients should not be pressured to accept treatment.

In the case of Ms B [51], an NHS Trust was held to have acted unlawfully for continuing to provide ventilation against the wishes of an adult patient with capacity. The Trust was criticised for not following the legal advice it had received and for allowing the situation to continue without taking immediate steps to address it.

Ms B

Ms B was a 43-year-old woman who, in the summer of 1999, experienced a haemorrhage into the spinal cord in her neck. She was admitted to hospital and a cavernoma was diagnosed, a condition caused by a malformation of blood vessels in the spinal cord. In February 2001 she suffered further damage to her spinal cord as a result of which she became tetraplegic, suffering complete paralysis from the neck down. In March 2001 Ms B asked for her ventilator to be switched off, a request that was repeated on many occasions. According to the medical evidence, without ventilation Ms B would have a less than 1% chance of breathing independently and death would almost certainly follow.

Although Ms B was examined by a number of psychiatrists and was deemed to have capacity, the doctors treating her refused to withdraw ventilation. They argued that her specific lack of knowledge and experience of exposure to a spinal rehabilitation unit meant that Ms B did not have the requisite information to give informed consent. The judge rejected this view which, she said, was not the law. The Trust was found to have treated Ms B unlawfully. Despite this the doctors involved were allowed to 'conscientiously object' to withdrawing the treatment and Ms B had to be moved to another hospital to have the treatment withdrawn. Ms B died in her sleep after ventilation was withdrawn.

Re B (adult: refusal of medical treatment) [52]

Health professionals can find it very difficult when a patient with capacity refuses treatment that they believe would provide a reasonable degree of recovery. While they may discuss their concern with patients, they must not put pressure on them to accept treatment. Ultimately the decision of whether to accept or reject the treatment offered rests with the patient.

25.6. The law on battery and assault applies equally where the patient is a pregnant woman and her refusal would put the life of the fetus at risk as well as her own.

A pregnant woman's right to refuse treatment was reaffirmed in the 1998 case of St George's Healthcare NHS Trust v. S [53] in which the Court held that adults with capacity have the *absolute* right to refuse medical treatment (in that case a Caesarean section) even if they may die as a result of that refusal.

In 2004 it was clarified that the Article 2 right to life in the Human Rights Act (see Section 18.3) does not extend to the unborn fetus and so the fact that a woman is pregnant does not affect her right to refuse treatment.

St George's Healthcare NHS Trust v. S

Ms S was 36 weeks pregnant and had not previously sought antenatal care. She was diagnosed with pre-eclampsia and was advised that she needed urgent attention, bed rest and admission to hospital for an induced delivery. Although she understood that without this treatment both her life and that of the fetus were in danger, she rejected the advice, wanting her baby to be born naturally.

S was seen by an approved social worker and was admitted to hospital against her will for assessment under the Mental Health Act 1983. An application was made to the court, and was granted, to dispense with the need for consent for the Caesarean section. Shortly afterwards her detention under the Mental Health Act was terminated.

Ms S appealed against the original judgment. Upholding the appeal, the Court of Appeal held that an unborn child is not a separate person and its need for medical assistance cannot prevail over the woman's rights. Therefore Ms S was entitled not to be forced to submit to an invasion of her body against her will, whether her own life or that of her unborn child depended upon it. The Court of Appeal also held that the Mental Health Act could not be used to detain an individual simply because her thinking was contrary to the views of most other people.

St George's Healthcare NHS Trust v. S [54]

25.7. Adult patients with capacity are entitled to refuse artificial nutrition and/or hydration and their refusals must be respected.

Although patients are not obliged to justify their decision to refuse ANH, health professionals should try to ensure that they have fully understood their situation and are not under any misapprehension about the nature of the treatment or the implications of their refusal.

25.8. Adult patients may, when they have capacity, make an advance decision setting out their wishes for treatment once capacity is lost (see Sections 28, 32 and 35). In England, Scotland and Wales competent adults may also choose to appoint a welfare attorney to make decisions on their behalf if they lack capacity in the future (see Sections 27 and 31).

Increasingly patients are taking a more active role in their own health care and have clear views about what treatment they would or would not wish to be given. Many people fear that once they become incapable of making decisions, life-prolonging treatment may continue to be provided long after it is able to deliver a level of recovery, or length and quality of life, they would find acceptable. Some people choose to express their views in the form of an advance decision refusing some forms of life-prolonging treatment. Information about the criteria for validity of advance decisions is given in Sections 28 and 32. Those considering making a formal advance decision should be aware of their disadvantages, as well as the benefits. In some parts of the UK competent adults are also able to plan for their future health care by appointing someone to make health care decisions on their behalf once competence is lost (see Sections 27 and 31).

Summary – Adults with capacity

- *There is a legal presumption that adults have capacity unless there is evidence to the contrary*
- *Health teams are not required to offer treatment that is clinically inappropriate*
- *Where a patient with capacity requests life-prolonging treatment that is able to achieve its physiological aim, there is an expectation that the treatment will be provided*
- *If a patient with capacity refuses life-prolonging treatment then that refusal must be respected*
- *Requests for, or refusals of, artificial nutrition or hydration by patients with capacity should be respected*
- *Patients with capacity may plan for future care by making an advance decision or, in England, Wales and Scotland, by appointing a welfare attorney*

---

26. Communication and information

26.1. Good communication and information is essential to decision making.

In order to make informed decisions, patients need to be given sufficient accurate information in a way they can understand (see Section 20.1). This will include information about the risks, benefits, side-effects, likelihood of success and level of anticipated improvement if treatment is given, the likely outcome if treatment is withheld and any other alternatives that might be considered.

26.2. Patients with capacity should be encouraged to be involved in decision making to the extent with which they feel comfortable.

While it is the role of doctors to advise about treatment and to decide what treatment options should be offered, it is essential that patients are given the opportunity to express preferences and to discuss their own wishes about treatment. Some patients may, for example, prefer a course of treatment that does not necessarily give the best clinical outcome but is more compatible with their lifestyle and values. In such cases patients' personal interests should usually take precedence over their strictly medical interests. Similarly, pain relief and sedation can sometimes reduce patients' overall level of awareness. Some people choose to tolerate a degree of pain in order to remain more alert.

26.3. Efforts should be made to comply with reasonable requests by patients with capacity about the provision of life-prolonging treatment.

The decision as to what treatment to offer rests with the clinician in charge of the patient's care taking account of input from other members of the health care team as well as the resource needs of different patients (see Section 17). Whilst it is not acceptable to continue to provide indefinitely treatment that is not clinically indicated and which seriously disadvantages other patients who have a better chance of survival, there may be arguments for complying with requests from patients with capacity for treatment to be continued or provided for a limited period.

26.4. Patients refusing medical treatment should have been offered information about the treatment proposed, the consequences of not having the treatment and any alternative forms of treatment available.

Patients refusing medical treatment should ideally base their decisions on sufficient accurate information including an awareness of the condition, the proposed treatment, any significant risks or side-effects, the probability of a successful recovery, the consequences of not having the treatment and any alternative forms of treatment. Such information should always be offered but, legally, patients are not required to have accepted the offer of information in order for their refusal to be valid [55].

Summary – Communication and information

• *Patients with capacity should be given sufficient information to make an informed decision and should be encouraged to be involved in decision making*

- *Patients' preferences about treatment options should form a central part of deciding care plans*
- *Efforts should be made to comply with reasonable requests from patients about the provision of life-prolonging treatment*
- *Although health professionals may find it difficult when patients refuse treatment, the decision of whether to accept or reject the treatment offered rests with the patient*

Part 6 **Decision making on behalf of adults who lack capacity**

Although the legal structures for decision making on behalf of adults lacking capacity differ throughout the UK, the same general principles apply:
- patients should be involved to the greatest extent possible;
- decisions should take account of the patient's wishes where they are known;
- where the patient's wishes are not known, decisions should be made in the patient's best interests; and
- those close to or representing the patient should be consulted.

This part of the guidance sets out the law in each jurisdiction within the UK and gives general guidance about the process of decision making including the key roles of consultation and communication. There is a particular risk that decisions to withhold or withdraw life-prolonging treatment from patients who lack capacity could be perceived as discriminatory (see Section 19). It is therefore essential that each decision is not only well thought through and based on the individual facts of the case but that the reason for the decision is clearly articulated, recorded and explained to those with an interest in the patient's care.

ENGLAND AND WALES

27. Patients with a Lasting Power of Attorney (LPA)

At the time of writing the Mental Capacity Act was due to come into force in 2007, putting on a statutory footing the legal basis for interventions in relation to adults who lack capacity to make decisions for themselves. For the first time in England and Wales welfare attorneys could be appointed to take decisions on behalf of adult patients once their capacity is lost. For doctors treating patients with a welfare attorney, this represented a significant change to their practice. The Act also creates a new offence of ill treatment or neglect of someone who lacks capacity. For more information on the Mental Capacity Act see the BMA's separate guidance [56].

27.1. In England and Wales an adult (over 18) with capacity may appoint a welfare attorney to give or withhold consent to medical treatment on his or her behalf once capacity is lost.

The Mental Capacity Act allows patients, while possessing capacity, to make a personal welfare lasting power of attorney (LPA) appointing a welfare attorney to make health and personal welfare decisions on their behalf once capacity is lost. Where an attorney has been appointed with the authority to make medical decisions, he or she must be consulted and give consent before treatment is provided (except in emergency situations where time does not permit such consultation). When acting under an LPA, welfare attorneys are bound by the general principles of the Act which are that:

- a person must be assumed to have capacity unless it is established that he or she lacks capacity;
- a person is not to be treated as unable to make a decision unless all practical steps to help him or her to do so have been taken without success;
- a person is not to be treated as unable to make a decision merely because he or she makes an unwise decision;
- an act done, or decision made, under this Act for or on behalf of a person who lacks capacity must be done, or made in his or her best interests (see Section 9);
- before the act is done, or the decision is made, it must be clear that the result cannot be as effectively achieved in a way that is less restrictive of the person's rights and freedom of action [57].

27.2. Although health teams should be aware of the possibility that a patient who lacks capacity may have appointed a welfare attorney and should make such reasonable enquiries as time permits, treatment should not be delayed where there is no evidence that an LPA exists. Emergency treatment should be provided while an LPA is being located or checks are made about its validity.

A register of LPAs is held by the Office of the Public Guardian (see Appendix 1). In addition, the Public Guardian can provide advice and guidance about the Act as well as dealing with any concerns about the way in which an LPA is operating.

Before the health care team relies on the consent or refusal of life-prolonging treatment by an appointed welfare attorney, they must be satisfied that:

- the patient lacks capacity to make the decision for him or herself;
- the scope of the LPA includes authorisation for the welfare attorney to make the decisions that are required;
- a statement has been included in the LPA specifically authorising the welfare attorney to make decisions relating to life-prolonging treatment;
- the LPA has been registered with the Office of the Public Guardian;
- the decision being made by the attorney is in the patient's best interests.

If a patient has not made a welfare LPA but has made a property and affairs LPA, the Mental Capacity Act Code of Practice recommends that this attorney should be consulted about health care decisions (wherever appropriate and practicable to do so) even though the attorney's decisions in relation to medical care will have no legal status [58]. Where these attorneys have known the patient for some time they may be able to contribute information about the patient's wishes and values to assist in determining best interests (see Sections 9 and 40).

27.3. Where there is disagreement between the health care team and an appointed welfare attorney or those close to or representing the patient about what represents the patient's best interest that cannot be resolved, the Court of Protection can be asked to make a declaration or it can appoint a deputy to make ongoing health care decisions on the patient's behalf.

Dealing with disagreement is discussed in Section 41. Information on how to make an application to the Court of Protection can be found in the Mental Capacity Act Code of Practice.

Where the Court of Protection has appointed a deputy this person must be consulted about health care decisions except where treatment is immediately necessary such that consultation is not practicable. Where there is disagreement between doctors and deputies that cannot be resolved by discussion and a second clinical opinion, the Court of Protection should be asked for a ruling.

Summary – Patients with an LPA

- *If the patient has appointed a welfare attorney with authority to make medical decisions, this person must be consulted and give consent before treatment is provided (except in an emergency situation)*
- *The authority of welfare attorneys only extends to life-prolonging treatment if that is specifically stated in the LPA*
- *Where there is disagreement about best interests the Court of Protection may be asked to make a declaration or may appoint a deputy to make ongoing decisions about medical treatment*

---

28. Patients with an advance decision about medical treatment

28.1. Where a patient has lost the capacity to make a decision but has a valid advance decision refusing life-prolonging treatment (including artificial nutrition or hydration) this must be respected.

Under the Mental Capacity Act doctors are required, by law, to respect a valid advance decision refusing medical treatment [59]. A refusal of a particular life-prolonging treatment does not imply a refusal of all treatment and, unless specifically refused, appropriate palliative care should be provided. Advance decisions refusing certain elements of basic care (see Section 11), including the offer of oral nutrition and hydration, are not binding on health professionals [60] and all procedures which are solely or primarily intended to keep the patient comfortable should continue to be offered.

Although health teams should be aware of the possibility that a patient may have made an advance decision, immediately necessary treatment should not be delayed in order to look for an advance decision if there is no clear indication that one exists.

28.2. In order for an advance decision refusing treatment to be valid (and therefore binding on the health care team) certain criteria must be met. Advance decisions that do not meet these criteria should nonetheless be taken into consideration in assessing the patient's best interests (see Sections 9 and 40).

An advance decision refusing treatment will be binding if:
- the person making the advance decision was aged 18 years or older when it was made;
- the person had capacity when the advance decision was made;
- the advance decision sets out the specific treatments to be refused and the circumstances in which the refusal is to apply;
- the advance decision has not been withdrawn;
- the person making the advance decision has not appointed, after it was made, an attorney to make the specified decision;
- the person making the advance decision has not done anything clearly inconsistent with its terms; and
- the individual lacks capacity to make contemporaneous decisions at the time the advance decision is invoked.

In addition, where the refusal applies to life-prolonging treatment, the advance decision:
- must be in writing;
- must be signed;
- must be witnessed; and
- must contain a signed and witnessed statement that it is to apply even where life is at risk.

Additional information can be found in the Mental Capacity Act Code of Practice.

In many cases it is impossible for a health team faced with an adult who lacks capacity with an advance decision to say with certainty that the patient had capacity at the time the decision was made. Equally, however, it would be wrong to always presume that an individual refusing treatment lacked the capacity to make that decision. As with contemporaneous decisions, there should be a presumption of capacity unless there are grounds to suspect otherwise. If, however, there are legitimate reasons to suspect that the patient may have lacked capacity – such as a history of depression, an underlying condition that might affect capacity, such as Alzheimer's disease, or if the family or friends suggest the patient lacked capacity at the time – immediate treatment should be provided to stabilise the patient whilst further enquiries are made. The fact that an advance decision was witnessed by a health professional should not be interpreted as evidence of capacity unless the witness has explicitly stated that the patient had capacity at the time.

28.3. Doctors faced with an advance decision should use their professional judgement to assess its validity.

The Mental Capacity Act has given some guidance about the type of factors that would invalidate an advance decision to refuse treatment. It states that an advance decision is not valid if:
• the person has withdrawn the decision while still having the capacity to do so;
• after making the advance decision, the person appointed a welfare attorney to give or refuse consent to the treatment specified in the advance decision;
• the person has done something that is clearly inconsistent with the advance decision indicating a change of mind [61].

Health professionals must use their professional judgement to assess whether the advance decision is applicable in the circumstances that have arisen. Particular care will be needed where the advance decision has not been regularly reviewed or updated and attention should be given to any changes in the patient's personal circumstances or in medical treatment since the decision was made. Where time permits, further enquiries should be made to establish the validity of the document and to help to clarify the patient's intentions, for example, by speaking to those close to the patient and contacting the patient's general practitioner. The Act gives some general guidance on the applicability of advance decisions, stating that an advance decision will not be applicable to the treatment in question if:
• the proposed treatment is not the treatment specified in the advance decision;
• the circumstances are different from any set out in the advance decision;
• there are reasonable grounds for believing that circumstances have arisen which were not anticipated when the advance decision was made and which

would have affected the advance decision had the person anticipated them at the time [62].

If the advance decision to refuse treatment is not applicable to the circumstances, it is not legally binding although it may still give valuable information about the individual's former wishes and values which can assist with determining best interests (see Sections 9 and 40).

28.4. Where there is genuine doubt about the validity of an advance decision and time permits, further enquiries should be made and, if necessary, an application may be made to the Court of Protection for a declaration. In an emergency situation, where there is no time to investigate further, the presumption should be in favour of providing life-prolonging treatment.

Although the Mental Capacity Act appears to give more scope for the advance wishes of patients to be respected, it remains to be seen how their implementation will be handled by the Court of Protection where there is any doubt about validity. Even before this Act, advance decisions to refuse treatment were binding under common law but in the few cases that were taken to court, the courts appeared to display some reluctance in declaring them valid and appeared to set a very high standard for them to be followed (see, for example, the case of KH in Section 29.4). In Re T (see Section 32.2), Munby J said:

> 'Where, as here, life is at stake, the evidence must be scrutinised with especial care. The continuing validity and applicability of the advance directive must be clearly established by convincing and inherently reliable evidence.' [63]

Recent evidence of the patient's wishes is therefore important. In one of the cases where the courts upheld the validity of an advance decision, the patient (AK), a 19-year-old man who had motor neurone disease, had made the decision just 2 weeks before losing all ability to communicate. In that case Hughes J held that:

> 'In the present case the expressions of AK's decision are recent and are made not on any hypothetical basis but in the fullest possible knowledge of impending reality. I am satisfied that they genuinely represent his considered wishes and should be treated as such.' [64]

28.5. Those close to the patient may be under the mistaken impression that they have the power to override an advance decision and health professionals complying with a valid advance decision should explain to the relatives their reasons for doing so.

Some advance decisions name an individual the patient would wish the health care team to consult in making treatment decisions. Unless this person has been formally appointed as a welfare attorney (see Section 27) the views of this person have no legal status and are not binding on the health care team. Nevertheless, given that the patient has asked health professionals to consult the named person, his or her reports of previous discussions with the patient are likely to provide information which is useful in determining whether and, if so, what treatment would be in the patient's best interests (see Sections 9 and 40). Responsibility for assessing best interests in such cases, however, rests with the clinician in charge of the patient's care.

28.6.   An advance decision requesting life-prolonging treatment (including artificial nutrition or hydration) should be seriously considered but there is no obligation to comply with such a request. Such statements should, however, be taken into account in assessing the patient's best interests.

The Mental Capacity Act Code of Practice advises that doctors must give 'special consideration' to written statements that ask for life-sustaining treatment (such as artificial nutrition and hydration) and that wherever possible all steps should be taken to prolong life. The Code acknowledges, however, that in some circumstances the provision of such treatment will be inappropriate such as in the final stages of a terminal illness or where the provision of ANH would cause great suffering and loss of dignity [65]. More common scenarios are where a patient has lost capacity in the final stages of life and providing artificial nutrition and/or hydration may prolong these final stages but at an adverse cost in terms of the patient's comfort and dignity, sometimes resulting in the patient's last days being spent in hospital rather than at home.

When considering the patient's best interests (see Section 9) the general spirit and tone of any advance decision should be taken into account as well as the actual wording of an advance decision requesting life-prolonging treatment.

Summary – Patients with an advance decision about medical treatment

- *A valid and applicable advance decision refusing treatment must be respected*
- *Where there is doubt about the validity of an advance decision, legal advice should be sought*
- *An advance decision requesting life-prolonging treatment should be carefully considered but there is no obligation to comply with such a request*

29. Patients without a Lasting Power of Attorney or advance decision

29.1. Where no welfare attorney or deputy has been appointed and there is no advance decision recorded, treatment may be provided to an adult lacking capacity provided the clinician in charge of the patient's care is satisfied that the treatment is in the patient's best interests (see Sections 9 and 40).

The Mental Capacity Act puts on a statutory footing the authority of health care staff to do what is reasonable and necessary to protect the health and well-being of an adult who lacks capacity. Before the Mental Capacity Act came into force this authority was covered by the common law and so, for those patients who have not appointed a welfare attorney and for whom there is no court-appointed deputy, the responsibility for decision making has not changed. An important part of the assessment of best interests is to discuss the patient's previously expressed views and wishes with those close to the patient. Where the patient does not have any family or friends, an Independent Mental Capacity Advocate (IMCA) must be consulted (see Section 29.3).

29.2. The same principle applies when decisions are taken in relation to a woman who is pregnant with a viable fetus and is unable to make or communicate decisions. The decision must represent the best interests of the pregnant woman.

The Article 2 right to life in the Human Rights Act (see Section 18) does not extend to the fetus and so any decision relating to a pregnant woman must be concerned only with her best interests and not those of the fetus. The extent to which the woman's own wishes about the outcome of the pregnancy may be taken into account in determining her best interests, however, is unclear. In order that these matters may be fully explored, legal advice should be sought.

29.3. Where the patient has no close relatives or friends to support them and the decision relates to 'serious medical treatment' an Independent Mental Capacity Advocate (IMCA) must be consulted.

The Mental Capacity Act set up the IMCA Service to provide representation and support for people who lack the capacity to make life-changing decisions and do not have anyone to speak on their behalf. It requires all NHS bodies or local authorities to ensure that an IMCA service is available.

It is a statutory requirement that an IMCA is consulted in every case where decisions are made about 'serious medical treatment' for this group of patients. Serious medical treatment is defined as treatment which involves:

> *providing, withholding or withholding treatment in circumstances where –*
> *(a) in a case where a single treatment is being proposed, there is a fine balance between its benefits to the patient and the burdens and risks it is likely to entail for him,*
> *(b) in a case where there is a choice of treatments, a decision as to which one to use is finely balanced, or*
> *(c) what is proposed would be likely to involve serious consequences for the patient [66].*

IMCAs cannot give consent on behalf of an adult who lacks capacity but they must be consulted and their views must be taken into consideration in assessing patients' best interests. Ultimately, however, the treatment decision rests with the clinician in charge of the patient's care.

More information about the IMCA service can be found in the Mental Capacity Act Code of Practice.

29.4. The courts have specified that declarations should be sought before withholding or withdrawing artificial nutrition and/or hydration from patients in persistent vegetative state (pvs) (see Section 30) but the same requirement has not been made for other patients who lack capacity. The BMA does not believe that non-pvs cases should routinely be subject to court review but, because particular care needs to be taken when making these decisions, the GMC requires that a second opinion is sought.

Decisions about ANH sometimes arise in connection with common conditions which currently are not taken to court but around which a body of practice has evolved. Such cases arise, for example, when elderly patients suffer from profound and irreversible dementia or have suffered a stroke which has left them similarly irreversibly brain damaged and both the family and the health care team believe that providing or continuing ANH would not be in the patient's best interests. In making such decisions, an assessment must be made in each case of whether the provision of ANH would provide a net benefit to the individual patient, taking account of both the benefits and the burdens of the treatment [67]. In the case of KH [68], the Court emphasised that an important factor to consider is the patient's awareness of his or her existence and surroundings and subsequent ability to experience pain or suffering as a result of the withholding or withdrawal of artificial nutrition or hydration. In practice, however, part of the responsibility of the health care team to all dying patients is to provide good quality end-of-life care including appropriate relief from any pain or other symptoms.

KH

KH was 59 years old and was diagnosed with multiple sclerosis in the mid-1970s. She had lived in a local nursing home for 10 years and had been fed by a PEG for 5 years. Most of her bodily functions had ceased to work, she was doubly incontinent, although conscious she could speak only odd words, was disorientated and did not recognise anybody, even her close family. She could, however, respond to simple instructions, such as sticking out her tongue on request and answer simple questions in a seemingly appropriate way such as when asked 'how are you?' she would say 'fine'.

In August 2004 her PEG fell out and she was admitted to hospital. All of the hospital staff wished to reinsert the PEG but the family unanimously objected to this. KH's brother, daughter and a close friend all argued that KH had made it clear, while she still had capacity, that she would not wish to be kept alive artificially if she was unable to recognise her children. In their view KH had no quality of life, experienced pain and suffering and would not want to be kept alive.

Mr Justice Coleridge ruled that the reported conversations with KH when she was competent did not meet the legal criteria for a valid advance refusal of treatment that was applicable in the circumstances that had arisen. The decision therefore had to be made on the basis of an assessment of KH's best interests. The patient was sufficiently conscious and sentient to experience the effects of withdrawing ANH over the period of time it would take her to die and the judge ruled that this would be even less dignified than the death she would face in the more distant future. He therefore concluded that withholding PEG feeding would not be in her best interests. The family appealed against the decision. The appeal was heard on the same day as the original hearing and the appeal was dismissed.

W Healthcare NHS Trust v. *H* [69]

In KH, Mr Justice Coleridge said: 'the Court cannot in effect sanction the death by starvation of a patient who is not in a pvs state other than with their clear and informed consent or where their condition is so intolerable as to be beyond doubt'. Reports of repeated conversations in the absence of other evidence were seen as insufficient indication of such consent. The emphasis in this case on 'intolerability' as being the touchstone of best interests relies on the original judgment in Burke v. GMC (see Section 5) and, referring to that case, Mr Justice Coleridge said: 'But for the recent case law, I would have refused the Trust's application'. Given that the case he was referring to was subsequently overturned on appeal and the specific parts of Mr Munby's judgment which appeared to give primacy to the notion of 'intolerability' was singled out for criticism, it is not evident that if this case was considered now, the same decision would be reached.

In KH, Mr Justice Coleridge referred to evidence from the barrister acting on behalf of the Trust stating that 'there has been no case in the books to date in which the court has sanctioned the withdrawal of treatment which is simply providing in effect the equivalent of food and drink for anybody other than somebody in a pvs state (in other words, someone who has no feeling of anything whatsoever)'. While it is true that no previous cases have been considered by the court it is, nevertheless, the case that ANH is sometimes withdrawn or withheld from patients who are not in pvs where this is agreed between all relevant parties as being in the patients' best interests. In the absence of any serious conflict of opinion or uncertainty about the patient's prognosis the BMA does not consider that all such decisions require legal review and no medical or legal body has suggested that legal review of routine practice in this area would be helpful. The fact that neither the judge nor the appeal court in KH suggested that these cases routinely need court approval adds weight to the view that where there is agreement between the health care team and the family or advocate about what is in the patient's best interests, court approval is not needed for the withdrawal of ANH from patients who are not in pvs. This interpretation of the law is also supported by the Mental Capacity Act Code of Practice which, in referring to cases that should be brought before a court, includes the withdrawal of ANH only where the patient is in pvs.

The BMA believes this is the right approach. ANH is not routinely started for all patients who are approaching the end of their lives, even if this could prolong their lives. This is because it is recognised that many people, at that stage, do not want to have that level of intervention and would feel that the burdens of the treatment outweighed the benefits. To take all of these cases to court would be disproportionate, expensive and distressing to all concerned. To distinguish between withholding and withdrawing ANH would also be unwise. If ANH could not be withdrawn, once started, without a court declaration, this may lead to a reluctance, among health care teams and those close to patients, to start it even though there may be some benefit. Greater protection can be afforded to patients by allowing health professionals and those close to or representing patients to decide where the patient's best interests lie, using established and agreed guidelines. It would be inappropriate for the courts to be expected to validate such decisions that have been made jointly by the health care team and those close to or representing the patient after careful assessment of all relevant factors. Rather, the court should remain as the final decision maker in the event of disagreement or where the patient's capacity, prognosis or best interests are in doubt.

Summary – Patients without an LPA or advance decision

- *Where no attorney has been appointed the clinician in charge of the patient's care must decide whether treatment would be in the patient's best interests*
- *Discussion should take place with the family or IMCA in assessing the patient's best interests*
- *Where there is disagreement about the patient's best interests legal advice should be sought*

---

30. Patients in persistent vegetative state (pvs)

30.1. Most treatment decisions for patients in pvs are made in the same way as decisions for other patients who lack capacity. The exception is decisions to withdraw artificial nutrition and/or hydration.

30.2. Proposals to withdraw artificial nutrition or hydration from patients who are in pvs, or in a state of very low awareness closely resembling pvs, and who are not imminently dying currently require legal review.

In 1993, the House of Lords concluded that it would not be unlawful to withdraw ANH from a patient, Tony Bland, who was in pvs (see Section 12). This was based on the view that ANH constituted medical treatment, the continued provision of which was not in his best interests. It was acknowledged at the time, however, that Bland's condition was very extreme and that in other cases where such action was proposed, the assessment of best interests may be less clear. In view of this and the very emotive nature of the withdrawal of ANH, the House of Lords recommended that, for the time being, in all cases where the withdrawal of ANH was being considered from a patient in pvs, a court declaration should be sought. It was clearly stated that this should be an interim measure until a body of experience had developed and other effective mechanisms for decision making had been put in place. As expertise and professional guidelines develop on pvs, the BMA can see no reason to differentiate between decisions for patients in pvs and those for patients with other very serious conditions where ANH is not considered to be a benefit, which are currently governed by established practice without the need for legal review (see Section 29). The BMA hopes that in future the courts will decide that pvs cases no longer inevitably require court review, where consensus exists, as long as such withdrawal is in accordance with agreed guidance.

At the current time, however, the clear advice from the English courts, and in the Mental Capacity Act Code of Practice, is that a declaration should be sought for each case in which it is proposed to withdraw ANH from a patient in pvs or a condition closely resembling pvs. (Since the current guidance states that the patient must have been in the condition for at least 6 months before a diagnosis of pvs can be confirmed, the question of *withholding* ANH from patients in this condition does not arise.) Whilst this advice is helpful in guiding and providing a degree of legal protection for health professionals, the legal effectiveness of such declarations has been questioned. A declaration from the court cannot make lawful a procedure which would otherwise be unlawful. If the action is lawful with the declaration, it would also be lawful without the declaration. The advantage of seeking such a declaration, however, is to assess, before the treatment is withdrawn, whether this action is considered to be reasonable in the particular case and to provide reassurance that all relevant factors have been considered. The withdrawal of ANH from a patient who is in pvs without a court declaration may be lawful but it would at present leave the doctor open to criticism, and potentially legal challenge, for failing to follow established procedures and guidelines.

In each case of patients in pvs that the courts have considered, it has been judged that it would not be unlawful to withdraw ANH. (By the end of September 2006, 36 such cases had been considered by the courts.) Some legal commentators have suggested that the inevitable conclusion to be reached from these cases is that ANH would never be in the best interests of a patient in pvs and should always be withdrawn. As stressed throughout this guidance, however, the BMA believes that such important decisions must be made only after very careful consideration of the individual circumstances in each case, rather than applying blanket decisions to certain categories of patients.

Summary – Patients in pvs

- *Most decisions for patients in pvs are made in the same way as decisions for other patients lacking capacity*
- *A court declaration should be sought before withdrawing ANH from patients in pvs*

SCOTLAND

31. Patients with a welfare power of attorney or welfare guardian

The Adults with Incapacity (Scotland) Act 2000 puts on a statutory footing the authority of health care staff to do what is reasonable and necessary to protect the health and well-being of an adult lacking capacity. It also makes provision for the appointment of health care proxies to make decisions on behalf of adults who lack capacity. For more information on the Adults with Incapacity (Scotland) Act see the BMA's separate guidance [70].

31.1. In Scotland a person with capacity over the age of 16 may appoint a welfare attorney to make decisions about medical treatment once capacity is lost. The sheriff court may appoint a welfare guardian with similar powers.

Where a welfare attorney or guardian has been appointed with the power to consent to treatment, he or she must be consulted (where reasonable and practicable) and consent to any proposed medical treatment. Attorneys may also refuse medical treatment, provided they are fulfilling their duty of care to the patient and are abiding by the general principles of the Act which include that any intervention must:
• benefit the adult;
• restrict the adult's freedom as little as possible while still achieving the desired benefit;
• take account of the adult's past and present wishes so far as they can be ascertained; and
• take account of the views of relevant others, so far as it is reasonable and practical to do so.
  It is important to note the first of these principles, that the Act requires any action taken to 'benefit' the patient. No definition of 'benefit' is provided although it is common in best interests judgements to accept that the patient's interests may be wider than purely providing medical benefit. If Scottish courts take the same position as their English colleagues, 'benefit' may be interpreted this widely but, in the absence of any ruling on this, doctors considering a course of action that is in the best interests of the patient but would provide no medical benefit would be well advised to seek legal advice.
  In addition to its clear proxy decision-making powers, the Act also requires doctors to take account of the views of the nearest relative and primary carer of the adult (with due regard to confidentiality).

31.2. Although health care teams should be aware of the possibility that a patient who lacks capacity may have appointed a welfare attorney or guardian and should make such reasonable enquiries as time permits, treatment should not be delayed where there is no evidence that one exists. It is important, however, before relying on the consent of a health care proxy to ensure that the attorney or guardian has the specific power to consent to treatment.

A register of valid proxy decision makers is held by the Public Guardian (see Appendix 1) and may be checked during office hours.

31.3. If the welfare attorney refuses to consent to the treatment proposed by the clinician in charge of the patient's care, that treatment can only be given following an opinion by a 'nominated medical practitioner' appointed by the Mental Welfare Commission for Scotland. This mechanism cannot be used if the doctor refuses to provide a treatment requested by the welfare attorney although where there is ongoing disagreement about whether treatment would benefit the patient an application may be made to the sheriff for a declaration.

Dealing with disagreement is discussed in Section 41.

Where the doctor nominated by the Mental Welfare Commission agrees that the treatment should be given, the treating doctor may provide treatment notwithstanding the disagreement of the attorney. Whatever the nominated doctor's opinion about the treatment, the treating doctor, welfare attorney or any other person with an interest in the personal welfare of the patient may apply to the Court of Session for a determination as to whether the proposed treatment should be given or not.

Summary – Patients with a welfare power of attorney or welfare guardian

- *If the patient has appointed a welfare attorney, or if the sheriff has appointed a welfare guardian, this person must be consulted if reasonable and practicable and must give consent before treatment is provided*
- *Where the welfare attorney or guardian refuses to consent, the Mental Welfare Commission must be asked to nominate a doctor to provide a second opinion before the treatment is given*

---

32. Patients with an advance decision about medical treatment

32.1. Advance decisions are not covered by statute in Scotland (except in relation to treatment for mental disorders) and nor have there been any specific cases considered by the Scottish courts. Nevertheless, the Code of Practice issued under the Adults with Incapacity (Scotland) Act states that advance refusals of treatment 'are potentially binding' [71].

The Scottish Executive, in its Code of Practice issued under the Adults with Incapacity (Scotland) Act, advises that a competently made advance statement

is a strong indication of a patient's wishes. In order to assess the status and validity of an advance statement, account needs to be taken of:
- the age of the statement;
- its relevance to the patient's current health care needs;
- medical progress since the statement was made which might affect the patient's attitude; and
- the patient's current wishes and feelings.

Given the emphasis in the legislation on respecting the known wishes of the individual, this statement in the Code of Practice and the Human Rights Act, it seems likely that a valid advance refusal of treatment, made by a patient with capacity, would be binding on health professionals. Until a specific case is considered by the Scottish courts, however, it is not possible to say, with certainty, how their legal status will be determined. Nevertheless, in other cases about withdrawing life-prolonging treatment, the Scottish courts have tended to take a similar approach to those in England and it is reasonable to assume that the same would apply in respect of the validity of advance decisions. This section therefore refers to the principles that emerged from the English cases as a guide for those working in Scotland.

32.2. In assessing the validity of advance decisions about medical treatment, it is likely, but not certain, that Scottish courts would take a similar approach to that adopted by the English courts before advance decisions were placed on a statutory footing.

It is clear from the cases that have been considered by courts in England [72] that an advance refusal will be legally binding if:
- the patient was an adult at the time the refusal was made;
- the patient had been offered sufficient, accurate information to make an informed decision;
- the circumstances that have arisen are those that were envisaged by the patient; and
- the patient was not subjected to undue influence in making the decision.

Re T

T was 20 years old and 34 weeks pregnant when she was injured in a road traffic accident. T's mother was a Jehovah's Witness but T herself was not. On two occasions, after spending time alone with her mother, T told staff she did not want a blood transfusion. A Caesarean section was carried out but the baby was stillborn. T's condition deteriorated and, had it not been for her advance refusal, the anaesthetist would have given her a blood transfusion. T's father and boyfriend challenged the validity of the advance refusal. The challenge was upheld and the blood transfusion was given. The basis for the decision was that T had been acting under the influence of her mother and the refusal did not represent a legitimate expression of T's free will. It also appeared that T had not been informed that a blood transfusion might be necessary in order to save her life and so it could not be assumed that she intended her refusal to apply to a situation that was life-threatening.

In dismissing the appeal against the decision, the Court of Appeal made clear that an anticipatory refusal, if clearly established and applicable in the circumstances, would be binding on health professionals. In T's case, however, these criteria were not met.

Re T (adult: refusal of medical treatment) [73]

32.3. The level of capacity required to refuse treatment in advance is the same level that would be required for making the decision contemporaneously.

It is irrelevant whether the refusal is contrary to the views of most other people or whether the patient lacks insight into other aspects of his or her life. The courts upheld, for example, the rights of a Broadmoor patient with a psychotic disorder to refuse amputation of his gangrenous foot even though he held demonstrably erroneous views on other matters [74].

Re C

C was a 68-year-old patient with paranoid schizophrenia. In 1993, during his confinement in a secure hospital, he developed gangrene in his foot. According to medical opinion there was an 85% chance that C would die if the leg was not amputated below the knee. Whilst content to follow medical advice and to co-operate with more conservative treatment, C refused to consent to the amputation.

C had grandiose and persecutory delusions, including that he had an international career in medicine. He expressed complete confidence in his ability to survive aided by God and the health care team but he acknowledged the possibility of death as a consequence of his refusal of amputation.

The High Court was asked to decide whether C had the capacity to make the decision. The Court held that although C's schizophrenia impacted on his general capacity, he was able to make a valid decision about the treatment. Therefore the amputation could not proceed without his consent and nor could it be carried out in the future if his mental capacity deteriorated.

Re C (adult: refusal of treatment) [75]

32.4. Where there is doubt about the validity or status of an advance refusal of treatment and time permits, legal advice should be sought. In an emergency situation, however, there should be a presumption in favour of life and emergency treatment should be provided.

Doctors must use their professional judgement to assess the validity of an advance refusal of treatment (see Sections 28.3 and 28.4).

32.5. Advance requests for life-prolonging treatment are not binding on health professionals but they should be carefully considered and assessed as part of the assessment of best interests.

Summary – Patients with an advance decision about medical treatment

- *A valid advance refusal of treatment is potentially binding on health professionals*
- *Where there is doubt about the status or validity of an advance refusal of treatment, legal advice should be sought*
- *Advance requests for life-prolonging treatment are not binding on health professionals but should be carefully considered as part of the assessment of best interests*

---

33. Patients without a welfare power of attorney or advance decision

33.1. In Scotland where no welfare attorney has been appointed, treatment may be provided to an adult lacking capacity provided the doctor in charge of the patient's care is satisfied that the treatment proposed is justified by reference to the principles of the Adults with Incapacity (Scotland) Act (see Section 31.1).

33.2. The same principle applies when decisions are taken in relation to a woman who is pregnant with a viable fetus and is unable to make or communicate decisions. The decision must be that which represents the best interests of the pregnant woman.

The Article 2 right to life in the Human Rights Act (see Section 18) does not extend to the fetus and so any decision relating to a pregnant woman must be concerned only with her best interests and not those of the fetus. The extent to which the woman's own wishes about the outcome of the pregnancy may be taken into account in determining her best interests, however, is unclear. In order that these matters may be fully explored, legal advice should be sought.

33.3. Where there is disagreement between the health care team and those close to the patient about what represents the patient's best interests, the sheriff can be asked to make a declaration or can appoint a welfare guardian to make ongoing health care decisions on the patient's behalf.

Anybody claiming an interest in the welfare of the patient may appeal a decision on medical treatment to the sheriff. Unlike the situation where there is a welfare attorney or guardian, the doctor may administer treatment unless the sheriff makes an order that prohibits it. The party that objects to the decision could apply to be the adult's welfare guardian.

33.4. No legal guidance has been provided by the courts in Scotland on decisions to withhold or withdraw artificial nutrition or hydration from patients who are not in pvs and are not imminently dying. The BMA does not believe that such cases should routinely be subject to court review but, because particular care needs to be taken when making these decisions, the GMC requires that a second opinion is sought.

The BMA's view on this issue is discussed in Section 29.4.

Summary – Patients without a welfare power of attorney or advance decision

- *Where no attorney has been appointed the doctor in charge of the patient's care must decide whether treatment would be in line with the principles of incapacity legislation*
- *Where those close to the patient disagree with the health care team's decision about treatment, they can ask the sheriff to make a declaration about whether treatment should be provided and/or apply to be the welfare guardian*

---

34. Patients in persistent vegetative state (pvs)

34.1. Decisions taken on behalf of patients in pvs should be made in the same way as decisions for other patients who lack capacity.

34.2. In Scotland the withdrawal of artificial nutrition and hydration (ANH) from a patient in pvs does not require a court declaration.

Unlike in England (see Section 30), it is not necessary in Scotland to apply to the courts in every case where the withdrawal of artificial nutrition and/or hydration is proposed from a patient in pvs [76]. The Court of Session has confirmed its authority to consider such cases but did not make such consideration a formal requirement. The Lord Advocate further indicated that, where such authority has been granted by the Court of Session, the doctor would not face prosecution. This leaves open the possibility of prosecution should the doctor not seek authority from the Court of Session. Although a court declaration may not be necessary, some doctors or hospitals may prefer to seek this reassurance.

Summary – Patients in pvs

- *Decisions taken on behalf of patients in pvs should be made in the same way as decisions for other patients who lack capacity*

NORTHERN IRELAND

35. Patients with an advance decision about medical treatment

35.1. Advance decisions about medical treatment are not covered by statute in Northern Ireland and nor have there been any specific cases considered by the courts in Northern Ireland. It is likely that the courts in Northern Ireland would take a similar approach to the English courts which have established that a valid advance refusal of treatment has the same legal authority as a contemporaneous refusal [77].

The approach adopted by English courts before advance decisions were placed on a statutory footing is discussed in Sections 32.2–32.5.

36. Patients without an advance decision about medical treatment

36.1. At present in Northern Ireland nobody has the power to give or withhold consent for the treatment of an adult who lacks decision-making capacity but treatment may be provided, without consent, if it is considered by the clinician in charge of the patient's care to be necessary and in the best interests of the patient.

There is currently no statute in Northern Ireland concerning decision making for adults who lack capacity. At the time of writing, legislation for Northern Ireland, along the lines of the Mental Capacity Act, was planned but not imminent (up-to-date information can be found on the BMA's website at www.bma.org.uk/ethics). Until such legislation is in force, decisions about whether to provide, withhold or withdraw treatment are the responsibility of the treating clinician following consultation with the rest of the health care team and those close to the patient and with reference to the courts in particularly contentious, difficult or disputed cases.

The legal authority for treating adults who lack capacity without consent comes from the 1989 case of Re F [78] in which the Court clarified that treatment may be provided to an adult who lacked capacity where that treatment is necessary ('action properly taken to preserve the life, health or well-being of the assisted person') and in the patient's best interests. By its very nature, the provision of life-prolonging treatment will preserve the life of the patient but it may not be in the patient's best interests (see Section 9). Where the treatment is not benefiting the patient, in a broad sense, the justification for providing the treatment does not exist and treatment cannot lawfully be provided.

Re F

F was 36 years old and had a severe mental disorder. She was described in Court as having the verbal capacity of a 2 year old and the general mental capacity of a 4 or 5 year old. F had been a hospital inpatient for more than 20 years and over that period had made great progress such that she was given increased freedom within the confines of the hospital. Her mental capacity was not, however, expected to improve. Over time F had developed a sexual relationship with another patient. It was said that the psychiatric consequences for F of becoming pregnant would be 'catastrophic'. Consideration had been given to the option of preventing F from forming sexual relationships but the view was taken that this could be achieved only by seriously restricting her already limited freedom. Less invasive methods of contraception had been considered but none was suitable so an application was made for a declaration that it would not be unlawful to sterilise F despite her being unable to give consent. All parties were agreed that sterilisation would be in F's best interests but a number of legal issues needed to be resolved.

The House of Lords ruled that the common law allowed doctors to give medical or surgical treatment to an adult patient who is incapable of consenting when the treatment is necessary ('action properly taken to preserve the life, health or well-being of the assisted person') and in the patient's best interests. Where the treatment proposed was sterilisation for non-therapeutic purposes, however, it was recommended that an application should be made to the court in each case for a declaration on whether sterilisation would be in the best interests of the patient.

Re F (mental patient: sterilisation) [79]

Information about assessing best interests is provided in Sections 9 and 40.

36.2. The same principle applies when decisions are taken in relation to a woman who is pregnant with a viable fetus and is unable to make or communicate decisions. The decision must be that which represents the best interests of the pregnant woman.

The Article 2 right to life in the Human Rights Act (see Section 18) does not extend to the fetus and so any decision relating to a pregnant woman must be concerned only with her best interests and not those of the fetus. The extent to which the woman's own wishes about the outcome of the pregnancy may be taken into account in determining her best interests, however, is unclear. In order that these matters may be fully explored, legal advice should be sought.

36.3. Where there is disagreement between the health care team and those close to the patient about what represents the patient's best interests that cannot be resolved, legal advice should be sought.

Guidance on dealing with disagreement can be found in Section 41.

36.4. No legal guidance has been provided by the courts in Northern Ireland on decisions to withhold or withdraw artificial nutrition or hydration from patients who are not in pvs and are not imminently dying. The BMA does not believe that such cases should routinely be subject to court review but, because particular care needs to be taken when making these decisions, the GMC requires that a second opinion is sought.

The BMA's view on this issue is discussed in Section 29.4.

Summary – Patients without an advance decision about medical treatment

- *Nobody can consent to or refuse treatment on behalf of another adult*
- *Where patients lack capacity the clinician in charge of the patient's care must decide whether treatment would be in the patient's best interests*
- *Where there is disagreement between the health care team and those close to the patient that cannot be resolved legal advice should be sought*

---

37. Patients in persistent vegetative state (pvs)

37.1. Most treatment decisions for patients in pvs are made in the same way as decisions for other patients who lack capacity. The exception is decisions to withdraw ANH.

37.2. Proposals to withdraw artificial nutrition and hydration (ANH) from patients who are in pvs, or in a state of very low awareness closely resembling pvs, and who are not imminently dying currently require legal review.

The situation in Northern Ireland is the same as in England and Wales (see Section 30).

Summary – Patients in pvs

- *Most decisions for patients in pvs are made in the same way as decisions for other patients lacking capacity*
- *A court declaration should be sought before withdrawing ANH from patients in pvs*

ALL UK JURISDICTIONS

38. Capacity and incapacity

38.1. There is a legal presumption that adults have the capacity to make decisions unless the contrary is proven. Where there are grounds for doubting capacity further investigation is required.

38.2. People have varying levels of capacity and should be encouraged to participate in discussion and decision making about all aspects of their lives to the greatest extent possible. Greater evidence of capacity will be required for decisions that have implications that are potentially detrimental to the patient.

Capacity is often discussed as though it is something that patients either definitively have or lack but the boundary is often less certain. People have varying levels of capacity and an individual's capacity may fluctuate over time; some older patients, for example, have periods of confusion followed by periods of lucidity and care is needed to encourage discussion and participation as and when appropriate for that patient. Individuals should be given practical assistance to maximise their decision-making capacity. This should include providing information in broad terms and simple language, including material translated into other languages if appropriate, and other modes of communication such as video or audio cassette. Patients should not be regarded as incapable of making or communicating a decision unless all practical steps have been taken to maximise their ability to do so (see Section 20.1). For some patients, however, such as those with advanced dementia, in a coma or pvs, all decision-making capacity is clearly lacking.

Capacity is task specific so individuals may have the capacity to make some decisions but not others. The evidence of capacity required will depend upon the consequences of the decision being taken. Greater evidence of understanding and capacity will be required to refuse life-prolonging treatment than will be necessary, for example, to refuse a flu vaccination. Patients who have not attained the required level should still, where possible, be involved in discussion about treatment options even though their views may not be determinative.

Where there is genuine uncertainty about an individual's capacity to refuse life-prolonging treatment, advice should be sought from a psychiatrist or an appropriately experienced chartered clinical psychologist. Individuals are considered legally unable to make decisions for themselves where they are unable to:
- understand the information relevant to the decision;
- retain that information;
- use or weigh that information as part of the process of making the decision; or
- communicate the decision [80].

Guidance on assessing mental capacity can be found in the Mental Capacity Act Code of Practice.

Summary – Capacity and incapacity

- *There is a legal presumption that adults have the capacity to make decisions unless the contrary is proven*
- *Patients should not be regarded as incapable of making or communicating a decision unless all practical steps have been taken to maximise their ability to do so*
- *Greater evidence of capacity will be required for decisions that have serious implications*

---

39. Communication and information

39.1. Where patients have some level of understanding they should be provided with information in a way they can understand and encouraged to participate in discussion to the extent to which they are able (see Section 20.1).

39.2. Appointed welfare attorneys, whose authority extend to medical decisions, and court-appointed deputies have the right to give or withhold consent to treatment and so must be involved in making non-emergency treatment decisions.

Where, in England, Wales and Scotland, welfare attorneys have been appointed to make medical decisions on behalf of patients lacking capacity, all non-emergency treatment decisions should be discussed with them. The health care team must provide the attorney with all the relevant information to make the decision including the risks, benefits, side-effects, likelihood of success and level of anticipated improvement if treatment is given, the likely outcome if treatment is withheld and any other alternatives that might be considered. The health care team should also be prepared to help attorneys to think through the issues, encourage them to discuss the options with members of the health care team or with others close to the patient, if they feel this would help, and offer any advice or assistance they require to make the decision. Making decisions to withdraw treatment is difficult for all concerned and attorneys are likely to require help and support throughout and following the decision-making process.

39.3. Even where their views have no legal status in terms of actual decision making, those close to or representing the patient are often able to provide important information to help ascertain whether the patient would have considered life-prolonging treatment to be beneficial. When assessing best interests, therefore, the views of those close to the patient should be sought and taken into account.

It is a common misperception that the 'next of kin' has legal rights to be informed of, and consulted about, an individual's medical condition and treatment. In fact there is no such legal right. Unless an individual has appointed a welfare attorney, or the court has appointed a guardian or deputy, nobody can give consent on behalf of another adult and nobody has the right to information about the patient. Nevertheless, it is good practice to consult with those close to the patient where that is not contrary to the known wishes of an adult lacking capacity; where a decision to withhold or withdraw treatment is made principally on 'quality of life' considerations (see Section 6), this is essential. In the absence of any clear indication from the patient about who should be consulted, health professionals may find it helpful to look towards the hierarchy of relatives provided in the Human Tissue Act 2004 and the Human Tissue (Scotland) Act 2006. In order of priority in England, Wales

and Northern Ireland this is:
  (i) spouse or partner (including civil or same sex partner)
  (ii) parent or child
  (iii) brother or sister
  (iv) grandparent or grandchild
  (v) niece or nephew
  (vi) stepfather or stepmother
 (vii) half-brother or half-sister
(viii) friend of long-standing
  In Scotland the order is:
  (i) spouse or civil partner
  (ii) living as husband and wife or in a relationship similar to a civil partnership for at least 6 months
  (iii) child
  (iv) parent
  (v) brother or sister
  (vi) grandparent
 (vii) grandchild
(viii) uncle or aunt
  (ix) cousin
  (x) niece or nephew
  (xi) friend of long-standing

It is important to be clear when consulting those close to the patient that the information sought relates to any views the patient expressed, or views the patient held, when he or she had capacity that might help to ascertain what he or she would have wanted in these circumstances. It is not what those consulted would like for the patient or what they would want for themselves if they were in the same situation. In practice, the extent to which friends and relatives are able to provide this information is likely to be dependent upon whether the patient has discussed the issues with them. Knowing the patient, however, they may be able to give a clearer picture of the type of values the patient held and the things that were important to the patient when he or she had capacity.

39.4. Although important, seeking views from those close to a patient who has lost decision-making capacity, or the ability to communicate, is not unproblematic.

Studies have shown that relatives' perceptions of patients' likely views often differ substantially from those patients' own wishes [81]. Often, relatives

tend to have a more negative impression of the condition than the patient
him or herself but, on the other hand, they may not wish to see themselves
as responsible for the withholding of treatment and so insist the patient
would want the treatment to continue. There is also a risk that an 'off the
cuff' remark, made without careful consideration of the implications, may
be given inappropriate significance and taken as evidence of the individual's
wishes. Particular difficulties can arise where there is disagreement within
the family about what the patient would have wanted or where conflicting
information is given by relatives. Concern may also arise where the family may
be thought to have motives other than the patient's best interests. Recognising
these difficulties, however, seeking information from those close to the patient
presents the only opportunity for the health care team to gain any impression
of the patient's likely wishes and values as part of the assessment of best
interests. With appropriate regard for confidentiality, information should be
sought, wherever possible, from more than one person and great care is needed
in interpreting any information received, which should be seen as one part
of a wider decision-making process rather than necessarily being judged as
conclusive. Where the patient has appointed a welfare attorney, this person's
views will take precedence over those of other family members, unless these
views are contrary to the patient's best interests. Relatives and carers may need
varying degrees of support to come to terms with the decision made.

Health professionals are well aware that discussion with those close to the
patient about withholding or withdrawing life-prolonging treatment needs
sensitive handling. Time and thought need to be given to how partners, parents
and relatives can discuss the diagnosis, prognosis and treatment options in
an unpressured environment. It can sometimes be helpful to formalise such
discussions, as in a case conference, to include the main members of the health
care team and the people closest to the patient although some relatives find
such meetings intimidating.

**39.5. In talking to those close to the patient a balance must be sought
between preserving confidentiality and obtaining sufficient information
to make an informed assessment.**

Where patients have, when possessing capacity, expressed a specific wish that
their condition should not be discussed with relatives or friends, this should
be respected. This should not, however, prevent the health care team from
seeking information from them about the patient's wishes and values. In
addition to seeking information, discussing the issues with those close to the
patient can also help them to come to terms with the situation. It may be
useful, as part of this discussion, to emphasise that the health care team and

those close to the patient are all working towards the same aim – to benefit the patient – even if their views as to how that can best be achieved may differ.

It is essential that those consulted are absolutely clear about their legal status in relation to the treatment decision. Where those consulted have the legal right to give or withhold consent on behalf of the patient, this should be made clear. Where, however, their views are not binding but are part of a process of arriving at a best interests judgement, they should be informed that, ultimately, making the treatment decision is not their right or their responsibility.

39.6. In England and Wales, where patients have no close relatives or friends to support them and the decision relates to 'serious medical treatment' an IMCA must be consulted (see Section 29.3).

Summary – Communication and information

- *Where patients have some level of understanding they should be provided with information in a way they can understand*
- *Appointed welfare attorneys whose authority extends to medical decisions have the right to give or withhold consent to treatment and so must be involved in making non-emergency treatment decisions*
- *Where a decision to withhold or withdraw treatment is made principally on 'quality of life' considerations, this must be discussed with those close to or representing the patient*
- *In England and Wales, where patients have no close relatives or friends and the decision relates to 'serious medical treatment' an IMCA must be consulted*

---

40. Assessing best interests

40.1. The central question in relation to treatment decisions for patients who lack capacity is whether the particular treatment would be in the best interests of the patient (see Section 9). An important factor in making these decisions is whether patients are thought to be aware of their environment or of their own existence.

Where the patient is in a stable but profoundly impaired condition, with no prospect of any reasonable degree of improvement, and despite assistance appears to be unable to communicate, further investigations may be needed to assess factors such as the patient's level of self-awareness, awareness of others and the ability to intentionally interact with them. Adequate time, resources and facilities should be made available to permit a thorough assessment of the patient's condition. This is a specialised task and very great care is needed to ensure that this assessment has been thoroughly undertaken by professionals with expertise in an appropriate range of assessment techniques. For example, an experienced psychologist and speech therapist may be able to provide additional insights to those of the usual treating team. Steps should be taken to optimise the conditions for such assessments such as ensuring that the patient is well nourished, that the use of sedatives is kept to a minimum and that the patient's physical environment is conducive to the best possible assessment of his or her capabilities. Adequate time should be set aside for the assessment which should, ideally, be undertaken over a period by an experienced multidisciplinary team.

40.2. Where treatment is able to prolong the patient's life but there are doubts about whether it would provide overall benefit, the health care team and those close to or representing the patient should take account of the patient's past wishes, values and preferences in order to assess whether treatment would be in the patient's best interests.

The courts have made clear that decisions about the provision of treatment should be made on the basis of whether a particular treatment would confer a benefit on the patient, taking account of both medical factors and whether the treatment is able to provide a reasonable quality of life for the patient (see Section 6). Where the individual lacks capacity and has not made a formal advance decision (see Sections 28, 32 and 35), this involves taking account of any previously expressed views or preferences or the values that were important to the individual when he or she had capacity. Those who know the patient are best placed to consider these broader best interests and so their input into the decision is crucial. If, for example, the patient is known to have held the view that there is intrinsic value in being alive, then life-prolonging treatment would, in virtually all cases, provide a net benefit for that particular individual. Many people, however, do not take that view and have not discussed their views about life-prolonging treatment with family and friends. While knowledge of the patient's previous views is therefore unlikely to provide sufficient information to give a definitive answer unless supported by other evidence, it can be helpful as part of the broader decision-making process.

40.3. Where the patient has never attained even a minimal level of capacity, decision making is more difficult. In these cases the primary factor will be the clinical benefits and burdens of treatment.

Where the patient has never had capacity and has therefore been unable to express any views about the circumstances under which life-prolonging treatment might be refused, or to provide any indication of those aspects of life which are valued, health professionals must rely on other factors in making decisions such as the patient's level of awareness and ability to experience pleasure or pain and the burdens of treatment. It is important for the health care team to be constantly aware that the primary consideration is whether the treatment would be in the best interests of the patient, not whether the health care team, or the patient's relatives or carers, would wish to have treatment themselves in that situation. As with other patients, in deciding what treatment to offer the health care team must take account of the competing health care needs of different patients. Nevertheless, care should always be taken to ensure that such decisions are made on an individual basis and that no unjustifiable discrimination occurs (see Section 19).

40.4. All patients are entitled to the same quality of care and those who lack capacity should not be excluded from potentially beneficial treatment options solely by reason of their lack of capacity.

Existing guidelines and court judgments have insisted that non-treatment decisions for people who lack the ability to make or communicate decisions should be based on considerations of benefit to the patient and not cost. It is obvious, however, that money spent caring for irreversibly and severely brain-damaged patients is money which cannot be used to treat other patients (see Section 17). This is an issue which needs to be acknowledged and addressed on a national scale as part of the debate on rationing and prioritising of resources. The BMA is concerned that, in reality, cost factors probably have a disproportionate influence on decision making for this very vulnerable patient group and is also concerned that the lack of a clear societal consensus on this most vexed area may unfairly leave doctors open to criticism. While doctors are required to balance the competing health care needs of different individuals, they must be able to show that this has been done fairly and not on the basis of unjustifiable discrimination.

40.5. In deciding to withdraw or withhold treatment the person responsible for making the decision about best interests must not be motivated by a desire to bring about the patient's death.

This statement, which is included in the Mental Capacity Act 2005, should not be interpreted to mean that doctors or welfare attorneys are under an obligation to agree to the provision of life-sustaining treatment in all cases.

Rather, they must use their judgement to assess all relevant factors to decide whether the provision of life-prolonging treatment would be in the patient's best interests. In cases where treatment is not considered to be in the best interests of the patient, the motivation for withholding it must not be a desire to end the patient's life but rather to stop providing a medical intervention that is not indicated because it does not provide net benefit for the patient. The distinction between foresight and intention (see Section 14) is of crucial importance.

40.6. **Where there is an appointed welfare attorney, guardian or deputy, whose role extends to decisions about life-prolonging treatment, that person is responsible for deciding what would be in the patient's best interests. This decision can be challenged if the health care team or others close to the patient disagree with it.**

40.7. **Where there is no health care proxy or welfare attorney, it is for the clinician in charge of the patient's care to make an assessment of best interests and to decide whether treatment should be provided. This decision can be challenged if those close to or representing the patient or other members of the health care team disagree with it.**

Summary – Assessing best interests

- *Before making decisions, adequate time, resources and facilities should be made available to permit a thorough assessment of the patient's condition including whether the patient is thought to be aware of his or her environment or own existence*
- *Consulting with those close to or representing the patient and taking account of the patient's past wishes, values and preferences are important components of the assessment of best interests*
- *Decisions to withhold or withdraw treatment from people who lack the ability to make or communicate decisions should be based on considerations of benefit to the patient*

---

41. Dealing with disagreement

41.1. **Wherever possible, consensus should be sought amongst all those involved about whether life-prolonging treatment should be provided.**

Efforts should always be directed at reaching consensus about the provision of treatment both within the health care team and between the health care team and those close to or representing the patient. Conflict within the health care team is likely to undermine the confidence of relatives or advocates that the right decision is being made and needs careful management. Hospital managers have an obligation to ensure that conflict management strategies are in place, such as an external mediator, and that junior medical and nursing staff, as well as carers and people close to or representing the patient, can express any misgivings they have about the basis of the decisions made. Although formal complaints procedures already exist, some concerns may be resolvable by informal discussion. It is also important that nurses and other staff can air their views within the team without fear that it will jeopardise their career prospects.

41.2. In the event of disagreement about whether treatment should be provided, the issue should be addressed and where possible resolved, without delay. Frequently, differences can be resolved through discussion and the offer of a second clinical opinion. Where agreement cannot be reached legal advice should be sought and, in some cases, an application may be made to the Court of Protection (in England and Wales), the sheriff (in Scotland) or the High Court (in Northern Ireland) for a declaration.

The European Court of Human Rights criticised the doctors in the Glass case (see Section 47.8) for not taking steps to resolve the dispute between the health care team and the patient's family before a medical emergency arose. In that case, the health care team did not have legal authority to provide the treatment because neither a person with parental responsibility nor a court had given consent and the situation was not an emergency such that treatment without consent could lawfully be provided. With treatment decisions for adults, even where there is no legal obligation to go to court in the event of disagreement, it would be advisable, where other dispute resolution mechanisms have failed, to seek legal advice. A court declaration does not make lawful what would otherwise be unlawful but it does give a clear indication of where the patient's best interests lie and therefore protects the health care team from criticism in the event of a challenge.

Where the patient is an adult who lacks capacity and there is an appointed health care proxy or welfare attorney, the codes of practice issued under the Adults with Incapacity (Scotland) Act and the Mental Capacity Act set out clear procedures to follow in the event of dispute. These procedures should be followed.

Summary – Dealing with disagreement

- *In the event of disagreement about whether treatment should be provided, the issue should be addressed, and where possible resolved, without delay*
- *Where agreement cannot be reached legal advice should be sought*

Part 7 **Decision making by young people with capacity**

In some ways decision making by mature minors who have capacity is very similar to decision making for adults with capacity (see Part 5) since there is opportunity for discussion with patients about what treatments they would consider to be in their best interests. The main difference is that in England, Wales and Northern Ireland those with parental responsibility may give consent on behalf of young people, even where they themselves have refused treatment. The situation is rather different in Scotland where it is likely that this concurrent authority of young people, their parents and the courts does not apply. In Scotland it is more likely, although not certain, that a young person's view would be considered determinative. This section sets out the legal situation in the different UK jurisdictions and considers some issues that are common to all decisions relating to minors who have the capacity to make decisions.

42. The law in England, Wales and Northern Ireland

42.1. The consent of a 16 or 17 year old has the same legal status as that of an adult. Nevertheless, the ability of parents and the courts to override the refusal of young people until they reach the age of 18 means that the guidance given in this section should be used for decisions relating to 16 and 17 year olds with capacity.

42.2. Below the age of 16 young people may give valid consent regardless of age provided they have sufficient understanding of the proposed treatment.

The law states that provided young people have sufficient understanding and intelligence to enable them to understand fully what is proposed, their consent provides the necessary legal authorisation for treatment to go ahead [82]. It is not necessary to have parental consent in addition to that of the young person with capacity and, indeed, treatment may proceed against the wishes of the parents [83]. Young people should however be encouraged to involve their parents and others close to them in important decisions including those about the provision of life-prolonging treatment.

Gillick v. West Norfolk and Wisbech AHA

Mrs Gillick took her local health authority to court because it refused to assure her that her five daughters, all aged under 16, would not be given contraceptive advice and treatment without her knowledge and consent. The case followed the publication of a Department of Health and Social Security circular advising that doctors consulted at a family planning clinic by a young woman under 16 would not be acting unlawfully if they prescribed contraceptives, provided that they acted in good faith and to protect the young woman from the harmful effects of sexual intercourse. In seeking a declaration that this advice was unlawful, Mrs Gillick argued that a young girl's consent was legally ineffective and inconsistent with parental rights. She said that it was therefore necessary to involve the parents.

This argument was rejected by the House of Lords, where the majority opinion was that the relevant test was whether the young woman had acquired sufficient understanding and intelligence to enable her to understand fully what was proposed. If she had this level of understanding and did not want her parents involved, a doctor would not be acting unlawfully in giving advice and treatment.

Gillick v. West Norfolk and Wisbech AHA [84]

In English law, the presumption of capacity applies only to people over the age of 16 and those providing treatment to those under 16 must assess the patient's capacity and understanding in each case.

42.3. Treatment in a young person's best interests may proceed where there is consent from somebody authorised to give it: a young person with capacity, somebody with parental responsibility or a court.

If treatment is authorised solely by the young person's father, it is important to be aware that not all fathers have parental responsibility (see Section 47.3) and, where there is any doubt about his authority to make the decision, further enquiries should be made.

42.4. Although young people's wishes should always be discussed with them, the fact that a patient has requested a particular treatment does not mean that it must always be provided.

Doctors are not obliged to offer treatment that is clinically inappropriate and nor are they required to provide all possible treatment to prolong life. The extent of the health care team's duty of care is discussed in Section 5.

42.5.   Provided it is able to achieve its physiological aim, artificial nutrition and/or hydration should never be withdrawn or withheld from a young person with capacity who has expressed a wish to remain alive. The provision of artificial nutrition and hydration (ANH) in these circumstances will always provide a benefit for the patient.

In the case of Burke v. GMC (see Section 5) the Court of Appeal stated that where a patient with capacity requests ANH this must, in almost all circumstances, be provided. It is difficult to know how far the principles established in that case can be extrapolated to other life-prolonging treatments and other circumstances. If a young person with capacity requests any life-prolonging treatment (such as artificial ventilation) that is able to achieve its physiological aim, then the expectation would be that the treatment would be provided. The courts have not, however, specifically addressed the resource issues raised by the duty to prolong life where that is the patient's wish but, for doctors involved with providing care, these will be serious considerations (see Section 17).

Advance requests for life-prolonging treatment, including artificial nutrition or hydration, should be taken into consideration in assessing best interests but are not necessarily determinative.

42.6.   A refusal of treatment (including artificial nutrition or hydration) by a young person under the age of 18 may not be determinative and treatment may proceed with the consent of either someone with parental responsibility or a court.

Although young people with capacity can, in law, give valid consent to treatment, it does not necessarily follow that they have the same right to refuse treatment. The courts have made clear that they retain their right to give consent on behalf of a young person until he or she reaches the age of 18.

In 1991, Lord Donaldson said:

> '[a Gillick competent] child can consent, but if he or she declines to do so or refuses, consent can be given by someone else who has parental rights or responsibilities. The failure or refusal of the Gillick competent child is a very important factor in the doctor's decision whether or not to treat, but does not prevent the necessary consent being obtained from another competent source.' [85]

Many of the cases involving young people's refusals of treatment have dealt with extreme or particularly complex situations, where the treatment being proposed is life-saving, and where there have been doubts about capacity.

> **Re W**
>
> W was 16 years old and living in a specialist adolescent residential unit under local authority care. Her physical condition due to anorexia nervosa deteriorated to the extent that the authority wished to transfer her to a specialist hospital for treatment. W refused, wanting instead to stay where she was and to cure herself when she decided it was right to do so. The local authority applied to court to be allowed to move W and for authorisation that she could be given medical treatment without her consent if necessary.
>
> The judge in the High Court concluded that W had capacity to make a decision to refuse treatment but that the court could, in exercising its inherent jurisdiction, override a refusal of medical treatment by a young person with capacity if that was in her best interests.
>
> W appealed against the decision. Her condition deteriorated significantly and the Court of Appeal made an emergency order enabling her to be taken to and treated at a specialist hospital notwithstanding her lack of consent. In delivering its judgment the Court of Appeal held that the judge at first instance had been wrong to conclude that W had capacity because a desire not to be treated was symptomatic of anorexia nervosa. Nevertheless, the Court said that its inherent powers were theoretically limitless and that there was no doubt that it had the power to override the refusal of a minor with capacity.
>
> *Re W (a minor) (medical treatment)* [86]

Although W was found by the Court of Appeal to lack capacity, it was made clear that even if W had been deemed to have capacity, treatment would still have been authorised to proceed because it was in her best interests. It was stated in this case that a refusal of treatment by a young person up to the age of 18, even if that person was competent, could be overridden if consent was given by a parent or a court, provided that the treatment was in the young person's best interests.

In the second edition of this guidance we questioned whether this overriding of the wishes of a person under 18 who has capacity would be seen to be compatible with the Human Rights Act (see Section 18), particularly young people's right to security of the person (Article 5), respect for privacy (Article 8), freedom of conscience (Article 9) and non-discrimination in the enjoyment of these rights (Article 14). In 2003, however, the courts considered the case of a young man, who was nearly 17 years old and a devout Jehovah's Witness. Despite his clear refusal of a blood transfusion, which was supported by his parents, the Court granted an order permitting the use of blood products if that was necessary to save his life. There was no suggestion in the judgment that the young man lacked capacity. In making the order Mr Justice Johnson referred to a statement by Nolan LJ in Re W that: 'In general terms the present state of the law is that an individual who has reached the age of 18 is free to do with his life what he wishes, but it is the duty of the court to ensure so far as it can that children survive to attain that age' [87]. Interestingly, the judgment makes no reference to the Human Rights Act although it must be assumed that the Court believed that the decision was compliant with that legislation.

Re P

P was a 16-year-old Jehovah's Witness with an inherited condition called hypermobility syndrome, the symptoms of which include a tendency to bleed because of the fragility of the patient's blood vessels. The patient was admitted to hospital suffering what appeared to be a ruptured aorta and both the patient and his parents expressed their objection to any treatment using blood or blood products. The doctors acceded to these views because the operation that would be necessary to cure what was then a suspected ruptured aorta was dangerous and likely to be unsuccessful; a blood transfusion was therefore considered futile. The crisis passed but the problem was unresolved. The doctors envisaged that a similar crisis may occur in which the use of blood products could become necessary to save P's life. The hospital asked the Court to authorise the use of blood products, despite P's objections, should this become necessary.

There was no suggestion in the judgment that P lacked capacity to make the decision or that he was not fully aware of the consequences of his decision. Mr Justice Johnson said there were 'weighty and compelling reasons' not to make the order but, nonetheless, looking at P's best interests in the widest sense and mindful of the court's responsibility to ensure so far as it can that children survive to adulthood, he granted the order requested.

Re P (medical treatment: best interests) [88]

Subsequent legal developments suggest, however, that this case should not necessarily be taken as determinative of this issue and if another similar case arises, legal advice should be sought.

42.7. Since their refusals of treatment may not be determinative, the advance refusals of young people do not carry the same weight as the advance refusals of adults.

Although not binding on health professionals advance refusals of particular forms of treatment by young people can play an important part in the decision-making process by helping to determine the question of best interests which must govern decision making by parents or the courts.

42.8. Other than in an emergency situation, treatment must not be provided for a young person without the consent of someone entitled to give it – the young person, someone with parental responsibility or the court.

Doctors faced with a refusal of life-prolonging treatment by a minor with capacity should give careful consideration to the implications of the decision – including balancing the harm caused by overriding a young person's choice against the harm caused by failing to treat. Where agreement cannot be reached by discussion and the offer of a second opinion, legal advice should be sought. Although legally treatment could proceed with the consent of someone with parental responsibility, where the young person has capacity and does not agree with the proposed treatment, legal advice should be sought.

Summary – The law in England, Wales and Northern Ireland

- *The consent of a 16 or 17 year old has the same legal status as that of an adult*
- *A young person who has sufficient understanding of the proposed treatment may give valid consent regardless of age*
- *Health care teams are not required to offer treatment that is clinically inappropriate*
- *A young person's refusal of life-prolonging treatment may not be determinative and legal advice should be sought*
- *Non-emergency treatment must not be provided for a young person without the consent of someone entitled to give it – the young person, someone with parental responsibility or the court*

---

43. The law in Scotland

43.1. From the age of 16, the decision-making procedures for adults apply (see Part 5).

43.2. Young people under 16 may give valid consent regardless of their age provided they have sufficient understanding of the proposed treatment.

In Scotland young people are presumed to have capacity from the age of 16 but may give valid consent to treatment below that age if they are considered capable of understanding the nature and possible consequences of the procedure or treatment [89]. The law also provides that from the age of 12 a child should be presumed to be of sufficient age and maturity to 'form a view' [90]. Although the consent of a mature minor is sufficient authority to proceed with treatment, it is good practice to encourage young people to involve their parents in important decisions including those about life-prolonging treatment.

43.3. Although young people's wishes should always be discussed with them, the fact that a patient has requested a particular treatment does not mean that it must always be provided.

Doctors are not obliged to offer treatment that is clinically inappropriate and nor are they required to provide all possible treatment to prolong life where no significant long-term improvement can be achieved. The extent of the health care team's duty of care is discussed in Section 5.

43.4. Provided it is able to achieve its physiological aim, artificial nutrition and/or hydration should never be withdrawn or withheld from a young person with capacity who has expressed a wish to remain alive. The provision of ANH in these circumstances will always provide a benefit for the patient.

In the case of Burke v. GMC (see Section 5) the Court of Appeal stated that where a patient with capacity requests ANH this must, in almost all circumstances, be provided. It is difficult to know how far the principles established in that case can be extrapolated to other life-prolonging treatments and other circumstances. If a young person with capacity requests any life-prolonging treatment (such as artificial ventilation) that is able to achieve its physiological aim, then the expectation would be that the treatment would be provided. The courts have not, however, specifically addressed the resource issues raised by the duty to prolong life where that is the patient's wish but, for doctors involved with providing care, these will be serious considerations (see Section 17).

Advance requests for life-prolonging treatment, including artificial nutrition or hydration, should be taken into consideration in assessing best interests but are not necessarily determinative.

43.5. A refusal of treatment (including artificial nutrition or hydration) by a minor with capacity in Scotland is likely to be determinative but in such cases legal advice should be sought.

The Age of Legal Capacity (Scotland) Act 1991 and the Children (Scotland) Act 1995 provide that a person may act as a child's legal representative (for example, by giving consent to medical treatment) only if the child is not capable of doing so on his or her own behalf. Thus the concurrent authority of young people with capacity, their parents and courts to consent, which is present in English law (see Section 42.6), is absent in Scottish law.

There has been little case law on the interpretation of this matter and at the time of writing, only one case had been reported. In that case, the Court upheld the right of a 15-year-old boy with capacity to refuse medical treatment and confirmed that his mother's consent could not authorise the treatment. However, the medical treatment being proposed was for mental illness and the Court ordered that he could, and in this case should, be formally detained under Section 18 of the Mental Health (Scotland) Act 1984 to receive the treatment. If the proposed treatment had been for a condition that was not covered by mental health legislation, it appears that treatment could not have been authorised. The question of whether the Court itself could override his refusal was not directly addressed but from the reasoning given by the Court, it would seem that this would have been open to the same objections.

Houston

An application was made to the Glasgow Sheriff Court in respect of a 15-year-old patient with symptoms of a psychotic illness. He would not consent to treatment and also refused to stay in hospital. The doctors believed that he was capable of understanding the nature and possible consequences of treatment and therefore had the capacity to make decisions on these matters. The doctors also believed that the right to consent carried with it the right to refuse and that his consent could not be overridden by his mother's consent. Treatment could only be provided, without his consent therefore, if it fell within the scope of the Mental Health (Scotland) Act, section 18 of which permitted detention on the approval of a sheriff. The doctors, and the patient's mother, were reluctant to use the mental health legislation because of the stigma attached to a detention order.

The sheriff took the view that the decision of a young person with capacity could not be overruled by a parent. He concluded that logic demanded that, when a young person was declared to have capacity, the young person's decision took precedence over that of a parent. Furthermore, he considered that the Age of Legal Capacity (Scotland) Act covered refusal as well as consent to treatment. The sheriff granted the detention order allowing the patient to be treated compulsorily under mental health legislation.

Houston (applicant) [91]

Although the situation in Scotland appears to offer more autonomy to young people, it is still to be seen whether the courts will hold minors to have sufficient capacity to make the decision to refuse life-prolonging treatment. If, however, young people under 16 are deemed to have capacity, it seems likely that their decisions to refuse treatment cannot be overridden by either parents or courts. Until this point is tested in the courts, however, it cannot be regarded as settled and in cases of doubt, legal advice should be sought.

Summary – The law in Scotland

- *From the age of 16, the decision-making procedures for adults apply*
- *A young person under 16 who has sufficient understanding of the nature and consequences of the proposed treatment may give a valid consent regardless of age*
- *Health care teams are not required to offer treatment that is clinically inappropriate*
- *A refusal of life-prolonging treatment by a young person with capacity is likely to be determinative but this point is not settled and, in any cases of doubt, legal advice should be sought*

---

44. Assessing capacity

44.1. Under the age of 16 there is no presumption of capacity and so an assessment must be made in each case although in Scotland young people are presumed to be able to 'form a view' from the age of 12.

The assessment of capacity in young people must look at the individual's understanding of both the condition and the proposed treatment.

44.2. Capacity is task specific so young people may have the capacity to make some decisions but not others. Health care teams will wish to have greater evidence of capacity for those decisions that have serious consequences, such as the refusal of life-prolonging treatment.

Efforts should be made to maximise the decision-making capacity of young people, including providing information in broad terms and simple language and using other methods of communication such as video or audio cassette. As with adults, young people are considered legally unable to make decisions for themselves where they are unable to:
• understand the information relevant to the decision;
• retain that information;

- use or weigh that information as part of the process of making the decision; or
- communicate the decision [92].

The BMA has separate guidance on assessing the capacity of young people [93].

44.3. Young people can have high levels of maturity and understanding in relation to their illness and it is important not to pre-judge them according to age.

Young people who have lived with disability or ongoing treatment for a particular condition or have experienced people close to them suffering in a similar way often have a much higher level of understanding and insight than others who lack such personal experience. These factors should be taken into account in considering the capacity of young people to make decisions.

Summary – Assessing capacity

- *There is no presumption of capacity for those under the age of 16 and capacity must be assessed in each case (although in Scotland young people are presumed to able to 'form a view' from the age of 12)*
- *Efforts should be made to maximise the decision-making capacity of young people*
- *Greater evidence of capacity will be required for decisions that have serious implications*

---

45. Communicating with young people

45.1. It is essential that young people are given sufficient information to make informed decisions and that they are encouraged to participate in decision making to the extent to which they feel comfortable.

In order to make informed decisions, young people need to be given sufficient, accurate information in a way they can understand (see Section 20.1). They need to know the risks, benefits, side-effects, likelihood of success and level of anticipated improvement if treatment is given, the likely outcome if treatment is withheld and any other alternatives that might be considered. Guidance on best practice for communicating with children, their siblings and parents is available from the National Institute for Health and Clinical Excellence (NICE) [94].

The role of young people in determining what their interests are and whether treatment would provide a benefit for them increases as their maturity and ability to express views develop. They should always be encouraged and helped to understand the treatment and care they are receiving and to participate in decision making to the extent that they are willing and able to do so.

45.2. Even though they are not obliged to do so, young people should be encouraged to involve their parents in important decisions about life-prolonging treatment.

Treatment may lawfully be provided with only the consent of a young person provided he or she is considered to have sufficient understanding to make the decision. Nevertheless, health professionals will want to ensure that their patients have adequate practical, physical and emotional support during treatment, or once treatment is withdrawn, and so should always try to encourage young people to involve their parents in such decisions.

45.3. Even where they are not determinative, the views and wishes of young people are an essential component of treatment decisions and should, therefore, be given serious consideration at all stages of decision making.

Young people should be encouraged to be involved in decisions about their health care to a degree with which they are comfortable; as well as being good practice, the law also requires that their views are heard [95]. Information cannot be forced upon unwilling recipients but older children sometimes benefit from having their wishes heard without having to accept the full responsibility of decision making alone. Some may therefore choose to delegate decision making to someone with parental responsibility (see Section 47.3) or to their doctors but should still be involved in discussions to the extent that they wish to be.

As with other patients with capacity, if a young person refuses treatment, time should be taken to explore the reasons for this and to ensure that any misunderstandings are corrected. Doctors should also consider what impact complying with a young person's refusal would have on his or her longer term chances of survival, improvement or recovery. For example, young people who have had repeated chemotherapy which has not provided a significant improvement, and for whom there is uncertainty about the chance of achieving therapeutic benefit, may decide that they do not wish to repeat it. When deciding what is in young people's best interests, having weighed the likelihood of clinical success, such refusals may tip the balance in favour of withholding further treatments.

Doctors are reluctant to force young people to have treatment against their will, even where the treatment would be lawful. Clearly the imperative to provide treatment weakens as the benefit it provides is less critical or its likelihood of success is smaller. Where non-treatment would be life-threatening or postponement would lead to serious and permanent injury, the moral arguments for providing it against a young person's will are stronger than if the procedure proposed is optional or the consequences of not providing it are less grave.

In addition to being difficult to achieve in practice and in some circumstances unlawful, forcing young people to undergo treatment could be damaging to the young person's current and future relationship with health professionals and could undermine trust in the medical profession. Whilst such considerations may not be determinative, the effects of overriding the wishes of young people must be considered in any assessment of their best interests. Where treatment is to be provided without the young person's consent and contrary to his or her wishes, every effort should be made to encourage the patient to co-operate with the treatment. In some cases, however, in order to provide necessary, authorised treatment, the use of some restraint or force may be required [96]. The use of restraint should be proportionate and should be used only as a matter of last resort once other options for treatment have been explored.

45.4. Young people should be given information at an early stage if there is a possibility that their refusal may be overridden, for example if their parents give consent, if a court authorises treatment or if treatment could be provided under mental health legislation.

Where a court is to be asked to make a declaration about whether treatment should be provided, the young person should be advised of this and informed of how his or her views can be represented in the case.

Summary – Communicating with young people

- *Good communication and information is essential to decision making*
- *Even though they are not obliged to do so, young people should be encouraged to involve their parents in decision making*
- *Young people should be informed at an early stage if there is a possibility that their refusal may be overridden*

46. Dealing with disagreement

46.1. Where there is disagreement about whether to give or withhold treatment which cannot be resolved through discussion and the offer of a second opinion, legal advice should be sought and, in some cases, a court may be asked to decide whether treatment should be provided.

In most cases treatment decisions are reached through discussion and mutual agreement between the health care team, young people and, usually, their parents or guardians. Treatment may not, however, be provided without consent except in emergency situations and so where the health care team believe that treatment would be in the best interests of the young person but he or she refuses, it will be necessary to seek legal advice. Although in England, Wales and Northern Ireland treatment may proceed with the consent of someone with parental responsibility (see Section 47.3), the courts have clearly indicated that the views and wishes of a minor who has capacity should be taken very seriously and should not easily be overridden (see Section 42.6). Although in Scotland it appears that neither parents nor the courts can override the refusal of a minor with capacity, this has not been explicitly tested and so legal advice should be sought.

Summary – Dealing with disagreement

- *Even where their views are not determinative the views and wishes of young people should be seriously considered in reaching treatment decisions*
- *Where there is disagreement, legal advice should be sought*

Part 8 **Decision making for children and young people who lack capacity**

This part of the guidance relates to children who lack capacity because of their age (babies and young children) and those who lack capacity because of their disability or physical condition, for example those who are unconscious. The law regarding decision making for children and young people who lack capacity is the same throughout the UK. Where they do not have sufficient understanding to make decisions for themselves, those with parental responsibility have authority to give consent to treatment that is in the best interests of the child. This will usually be a joint decision between the health care team and the parents based on good quality information and communication. Difficulties can arise, however, where views differ about where the child or young person's best interests lie.

The Royal College of Paediatrics and Child Health also has guidance on decisions to withdraw treatment from children [97].

47. The law

47.1. From birth, babies have the same legal rights as any other person and decisions must be taken that are in their best interests.

From birth, all people have the right to expect appropriate care and decisions must be taken in their best interests. Enquiries to the BMA appear to indicate that some doctors consider that if parental agreement is obtained, they need not provide life-sustaining treatment for babies born with a severe impairment. In fact, such decisions are only appropriate where they reflect the child's best interests.

47.2. In England, Wales and Northern Ireland young people who lack capacity come within the decision-making procedures for children until the age of 18 and then transfer to the decision-making procedures for adults. In Scotland this shift happens at the age of 16.

This part of the guidance is relevant to young people up to the age of 18 who lack capacity in England, Wales and Northern Ireland. Where a young person who lacks capacity in Scotland reaches 16 years old, however, the procedures for adults (set out in Part 6) should be followed.

47.3. Those with parental responsibility for a child or young person who lacks capacity are legally entitled to give or withhold consent to treatment (including, in some cases, artificial nutrition or hydration, but see Section 47.4).

Not all fathers have parental responsibility. Both parents have parental responsibility if they were married at the time of the child's conception, or birth, or at some time after the child's birth. Neither parent loses parental responsibility if they divorce. If the parents were never married and the child was born before 1 December 2003 (in England and Wales), 15 April 2002 (in Northern Ireland) or 4 May 2006 (in Scotland) only the mother automatically has parental responsibility but fathers can apply for a parental responsibility order. After those dates, if the father was named on the birth certificate, he automatically acquires parental responsibility [98]. Where there is any doubt, enquiries should be made to ensure the father has parental responsibility before relying solely on his consent. Some same-sex couples will both hold parental responsibility for a child [99]; where there is doubt about who is eligible to give consent on behalf of a child, further enquiries should be made. In relation to any controversial treatment, caution should be exercised. Wherever possible all holders of parental responsibility should be consulted. In the event of disagreement, doctors should always seek legal advice and all holders of parental responsibility should also be given the opportunity to seek legal advice.

Mothers automatically gain parental responsibility irrespective of their age and so a mother who is herself a minor, but who has capacity to make decisions, is able to give consent on behalf of her child in the same way as older mothers.

47.4. In England, Wales and Northern Ireland where a child or young person is in a persistent vegetative state (pvs), any proposal to withdraw artificial nutrition and hydration (ANH) should be subject to legal review.

The principle that legal review is necessary before removing ANH from a patient in pvs (see Section 30) extends to children, including those whose parents agree to the course of action proposed.

47.5. Although parents' wishes about the treatment of their children should always be discussed with them, the fact that a parent has requested a particular treatment does not mean that it must always be provided.

Parents cannot insist upon treatment that the health care team considers inappropriate or where the burdens of the treatment clearly outweigh the benefits for the child or young person. Whilst it is entirely understandable for parents to want to prolong their child's life for as long possible, it is unacceptable to expose fatally ill children to all manner of painful, unproven or essentially futile treatments. The doctor's first duty is to the patient and in such cases the main task may involve helping the family to gain a realistic picture of the level of expected recovery.

47.6. The decisions of those with parental responsibility about whether to accept or refuse the treatments offered will usually be determinative unless they conflict with the interpretation of those providing care about the child or young person's best interests.

Parents and the health care team will usually reach agreement over what is best for a child or young person who lacks capacity. Their goal is the same – to benefit the patient – and in the vast majority of cases their views about how this can be achieved coincide. All reasonable options should be discussed with the parents, although the actual treatments offered will depend on the medical assessment of benefit. Where there is genuine uncertainty about which treatment option would be of most clinical benefit to the child or young person, parents are usually best placed and equipped to weigh this evidence and apply it to their child's own circumstances.

The authority of parents to make treatment decisions is not unlimited and only applies where the decision is in the best interests of the child or young person. Their authority is likely to be curtailed where the decision made would be contrary to the patient's interests. This might be the case where, for example, the treatment refused would provide a clear benefit to the child or young person, where the statistical chance of recovery is good or where the severity of the condition is not sufficient to justify withholding or withdrawing life-prolonging treatment.

47.7. If agreement cannot be reached legal advice should be sought.

If, despite discussion, agreement cannot be reached a second opinion should be sought. If there is still disagreement, ultimately a court should be asked to make a declaration about whether the provision of life-prolonging treatment would benefit the child or young person. If the child has been made a ward of court, a decision must not be made about withholding or withdrawing treatment without seeking authorisation from the court.

The court is required to make the welfare of the child its paramount consideration and guidance on what factors should be considered is given in the Children Act 1989 [100] and equivalent legislation in Scotland [101] and Northern Ireland [102]:

(a) *the ascertainable wishes and feelings of the child concerned (considered in the light of his age and understanding);*
(b) *his physical, emotional and educational needs;*
(c) *the likely effect on him of any change in his circumstances;*
(d) *his age, sex, background and any characteristics of his which the court considers relevant;*
(e) *any harm which he has suffered or is at risk of suffering; [and]*
(f) *how capable each of his parents, and any other person in relation to whom the court considers the question to be relevant, is of meeting his needs.*

In exceptional cases, the courts have been willing to authorise the withholding or withdrawing of life-prolonging treatment, against the parents' wishes, where it was considered that continued treatment would be contrary to the child's best interests. In 1997, for example, the High Court endorsed a doctor's decision to withhold artificial ventilation and refrain from resuscitating a 16-month-old girl with a very serious disease [103].

Baby C

C was a 16-month-old girl with spinal muscular atrophy type 1, a progressive disease that causes severe emaciation and disability. She was dependent on intermittent positive pressure ventilation. Her doctors sought authority from the High Court to withdraw the ventilation, and not to reinstate it or resuscitate C if she suffered further respiratory relapse. They maintained that further treatment would cause her increasing distress, could cause medical complications, and could do little more than delay death without significant alleviation of suffering.

The judge described C's parents as highly responsible orthodox Jews, who loved their daughter but who were unable to 'bring themselves to face the inevitable future'. The parents' religious beliefs prevented them from standing aside and watching a person die when an intervention could prolong that life. The doctor's treatment plan of withholding resuscitation and ventilation and providing palliative care was endorsed by the judge to 'ease the suffering of this little girl to allow her life to end peacefully'.

Re C (medical treatment) [104]

The courts do not always agree with medical advice however, when decisions depend on the quality of life rather than on the ability of the treatment to achieve its physiological aim. In 2006 the High Court agreed with the parents of Baby MB against the unanimous view of the medical team and rejected an application from the NHS Trust for the withdrawal of ventilation [105].

Baby MB

MB was 18 months old with spinal muscular atrophy type 1. The Court heard that except for some movement of his eyes and possible slight, but barely perceptible, movement of his eyebrows, corners of his mouth, thumb, toes and feet, he could not move. He could not breathe unaided and required positive pressure ventilation via an invasive endotracheal tube and was fed through a gastrostomy tube. There was no hope of any improvement in his condition and his condition would inevitably deteriorate. The regular interventions required to keep MB alive caused him discomfort, distress and in some cases pain. Although unable to express this in any meaningful way, his heart rate would suddenly rise, his eyebrow would moved slightly and sometimes he produced tears. The medical team, including 14 consultants, all agreed that to continue ventilation was contrary to MB's best interests.

   The parents argued that, despite his disability, MB was able to experience pleasure from his existence which outweighed the burdens and any discomfort or pain. They said he recognised them and his siblings and appeared to gain some pleasure from being with them and from watching certain DVDs or listening to music. In rejecting the NHS Trust's application to withdraw artificial ventilation, Mr Justice Holman said, 'I must proceed on the basis that M has age appropriate cognition, and does continue to have a relationship of value to him with his family, and does continue to gain other pleasures from touch, sight and sound'. He concluded: 'I do not consider that from one day to the next all the routine discomfort, distress and pain that the doctors describe . . . outweigh those benefits so that I can say that it is in his best interests that those benefits, and life itself, should immediately end. On the contrary, I positively consider that as his life does still have benefits, and is his life, it should be enabled to continue'.

An NHS Trust v. MB [106]

The courts have also upheld a parent's refusal of a liver transplant against the advice of doctors in the 1996 case of Re T [107]. The child had biliary atresia and the unanimous view of the medical team was that he would not live beyond two and a half without the transplant. It must be noted, however, that this was a very exceptional case and many legal commentators have questioned the court's assessment of best interests in that case. In a subsequent legal case

Lord Justice Thorpe said of the decision: 'the outcome of that appeal, denying a child life-prolonging surgery, is unique in our jurisprudence and is explained by the trial judge's erroneous focus on the reasonableness of the mother's rejection of medical opinion' [108].

The decisions in these cases involving children make clear the importance and impact of a broad understanding of best interests. These cases illustrate the validity and weight the courts have given to parents' assessment of their children's best interests whilst showing that their wishes will not always be followed. Where decisions are finely balanced and it is not clear what would be best for a child, the views of the parents will, however, usually be determinative. Lord Justice Waite summed this up, saying:

> 'the greater the scope for genuine debate between one view and another
> [about the best interests of the child], the stronger will be the inclination
> of the court to be influenced by a reflection that in the last analysis the
> best interests of every child include an expectation that difficult decisions
> affecting the length and quality of its life will be taken for it by the parent
> to whom its care has been entrusted by nature.' [109]

47.8. Other than in an emergency situation treatment must not be provided for a child or young person who lacks capacity without the consent of someone with parental responsibility or the court.

Where it is evident that there is disagreement, steps should be taken, without delay, to resolve any dispute including, if necessary, seeking a court declaration.

Glass v. United Kingdom

In March 2004, the European Court of Human Rights (ECHR) awarded Carol Glass and her son David compensation after doctors treated David contrary to his mother's wishes, without a court order.

Born in 1986, David Glass was severely mentally and physically disabled, requiring 24-hour care. In July 1998 after surgery to alleviate an upper respiratory tract obstruction, David became critically ill and was put on a ventilator. Doctors thought he was dying. His condition improved briefly and he returned home only to be readmitted a few days later when doctors discussed the option of morphine to alleviate his distress. His mother refused, believing it would compromise his chance of recovery. She also made clear that she wanted David resuscitated if his heart stopped. Relations between the family and the health care team had completely broken down to the extent that some members of the family were later prosecuted for physically attacking hospital staff. Although the doctor managing David's care noted the possible need for a court order in such cases of total disagreement, no order was sought and the morphine was provided without consent.

The Glass family argued that, when the dispute arose, the hospital should have involved the courts to clarify whether, despite his mother's objections, the treatment proposed was in David's best interests and that the doctors were wrong in believing the urgency of the case made that unnecessary. Although dismissed by UK courts, the ECHR held that David's Article 8 right to privacy, and in particular his right to physical integrity, had been breached. The Court said it was clear that there was a dispute over treatment before the situation reached crisis point and the UK courts should have been used to settle the dispute before an emergency situation arose.

Glass v. *United Kingdom* [110]

Summary – The law

- *From birth, babies have the same legal rights as any other person and decisions must be taken that are in their best interests*
- *In England, Wales and Northern Ireland young people who lack capacity come within the decision-making procedures for children until the age of 18 and then transfer to the decision-making procedures for adults. In Scotland this shift happens at the age of 16*
- *Health care teams are not required to offer treatment that is clinically inappropriate*
- *Those with parental responsibility are legally entitled to give or withhold consent to treatment*
- *The decisions of those with parental responsibility will usually be determinative unless they conflict with the child or young person's best interests*
- *If agreement cannot be reached legal review will be required*
- *Other than in emergency situations treatment must not be provided for a child or young person who lacks capacity without the consent of someone with parental responsibility or the court*

---

48. Duties owed to babies and children

48.1. The same ethical duties are owed to babies and young children as to older children and adults.

The high standards set for decision making on behalf of adults who lack capacity apply similarly to decisions in paediatric care. Although specific and important differences exist between adult and child patients, the ethical principles which underlie the provision or continuation of treatment, namely that it should only proceed where it would provide a net benefit to the patient, hold for all. There is, however, often perceived to be a difference between the ethical principles guiding treatment decisions for adults and children which can manifest itself either in a belief that treatment may be more easily withdrawn, particularly from newborns, or in the importance of striving to provide every possible form of treatment. Evidence from America, for example, suggests that 'clinicians frequently give young patients more chances to revive from and survive their illnesses than they offer to older, particularly elderly patients. Clinicians also seem more willing to impose greater burdens on children with fewer chances of success than on adults' [111].

Willingness to continue with treatment may reflect the fact that a decision to stop striving to maintain life is psychologically more difficult to make for children than adults or that outcomes may be less predictable for children due to a small evidence base from which to judge the likely outcome. The high profile case of Charlotte Wyatt [112] serves as a reminder of the difficulty of accurately assessing prognosis in seriously ill young children and the importance of keeping treatment decisions constantly under review. The developmental potential of children is also important and paediatricians will consider the quality of this potential for progression from lacking capacity to possessing capacity as a factor in decision making.

Charlotte Wyatt

Charlotte Wyatt was born in October 2003 at 26 weeks gestation. By October 2004 she had not left hospital. She had chronic respiratory and kidney problems coupled with profound brain damage that left her blind, deaf and incapable of voluntary movement or response. She demonstrably experienced pain but her doctors doubted that she was able to experience any pleasure. It was expected that during the winter of 2004 she would succumb to respiratory failure that would prove fatal and the unanimous view of her medical team was that, should this occur, it would not be in her best interests to provide artificial ventilation; Charlotte's parents disagreed. The High Court was told that a realistic likelihood of her surviving for 12 months was around 5%. The judge concluded that further invasive and aggressive treatment would be intolerable to Charlotte and should not be provided [113].

In January 2005 Charlotte's condition had visibly improved. The medical team acknowledged that there had been some improvements but said this did not change her underlying condition. More investigations into Charlotte's condition and prognosis were planned and her parents asked that the earlier judgment be stayed while these investigations took place. The judge refused [114]. A further application was made in March 2005 for the earlier judgment to be discharged. Charlotte had, unexpectedly, survived the winter and her condition had improved such that her oxygen requirement was 50% compared to 100% in October 2004, she was able to respond to loud noises and she was no longer under constant sedation. Nevertheless the judge found that there had been no change in her underlying condition and again refused the application [115]. Mr and Mrs Wyatt appealed against this decision but their appeal was dismissed [116].

When the case was reviewed again in October 2005 further improvements had been made and Charlotte had been able to leave hospital and visit her home on a couple of occasions. The court rescinded the earlier declaration [117]. Between then and February 2006, however, her condition markedly deteriorated. She had developed an aggressive viral infection and the health care team felt it likely that within a few hours intubation and ventilation would be required to keep her alive, treatment they considered would cause her unnecessary pain and would not be in her best interests. The court agreed and issued a declaration that it would be lawful to withhold intubation and ventilation [118]. Again, against medical expectations, Charlotte's condition improved.

At the time of writing, in September 2006, Charlotte Wyatt was, according to reports, continuing to improve.

Portsmouth NHS Trust v. Wyatt [119]

Summary – Duties owed to babies and children

- *The same ethical duties are owed to babies and young children as to older children and adults and decisions must be taken on the basis of best interests*

---

49. Communicating with parents

49.1. It is essential that parents are given sufficient accurate information to be able to make an informed decision and that there is ongoing communication throughout the decision-making process.

The health care team must provide the parents of a sick baby, child or young person who lacks capacity with all the relevant information they need to make appropriate decisions (see Section 20.1). This should include the risks, benefits, side-effects, likelihood of success and level of anticipated improvement if treatment is given, the likely outcome if treatment is withheld and any other alternatives that might be considered. Where there is clinical uncertainty about whether specific treatments should be considered, because it is unclear whether they provide sufficient benefit to outweigh the burdens, parents should be informed of that in a frank but sensitive way. Parents are generally the best judges of their children's interests but they need full, clear and accurate information in order to make that assessment. Doctors and informed parents usually share treatment decisions, with doctors taking the lead in judging the clinical factors and parents taking the lead on determining best interests more generally.

Wherever possible, decisions should be taken at a pace that is comfortable to those involved, allowing time for discussion, explanation and reflection so that decisions are informed and reflective of the child or young person's best interests and so the parents have time to consult others close to them and adjust to their decisions. It may be useful to bring in additional clinical expertise and to seek further medical opinions and parents may benefit from the opportunity to speak with others who have been through similar experiences. Parents should also be given as much help and support as they need to make the decision.

49.2. Although parents who do not have parental responsibility do not have the legal authority to give consent on behalf of their children, they may, nonetheless, have a right (under the Human Rights Act) to be consulted and involved in decision making.

Where parents who do not have parental responsibility wish to be involved in discussion and decision making, this should be encouraged.

49.3. Young children and those who have disabilities that impair their decision-making capacity may be able to understand and contribute to discussions about some aspects of their care. Communication with children needs to be appropriate to both their age, development and level of understanding.

Children with insufficient maturity, understanding or capacity to make treatment decisions for themselves are often able to express views or opinions about their care. Ideally children and young people should be encouraged to talk about what is happening to them, so that they are given the opportunity to understand their illness and treatment. Their preferences on issues such as when to receive treatment, and where, should be taken into account and should influence decisions whenever possible. Children and young people who lack capacity to make decisions can also be encouraged to feel involved by allowing them to take other, easier, decisions, such as who should accompany them during treatment.

> *Summary – Communicating with parents*
>
> - *Good communication and information is essential to decision making*
> - *Parents without parental responsibility should be encouraged to be involved in discussion and decision making even though they may not, legally, give consent on behalf of the child*
> - *Communication with children and young people needs to be appropriate to their age, development and level of understanding*

50. Assessing best interests

50.1. The child or young person's best interests (see Section 9) and an assessment of the benefits and burdens of treatment are the key factors in considering whether treatment should be provided or withdrawn.

The BMA's guidance emphasises that where there is reasonable uncertainty about the benefit of life-prolonging treatment, there should be a presumption in favour of initiating it, although there are circumstances in which active intervention (other than basic care) would not be appropriate since best interests are not synonymous with prolongation of life. Criteria for deciding best interests are the same as those for adults who lack capacity (see Section 9), including whether the child or young person has the potential to develop awareness, the ability to interact and the capacity for self-directed action and whether he or she will experience severe unavoidable pain and distress.

If the child or young person's condition is incompatible with survival or where there is a consensus that the condition is so severe that treatment would not provide a benefit, in terms of being able to restore or maintain health, intervention may be unjustified. Similarly, where treatments would involve suffering or distress to the child or young person, these and other burdens must be weighed against the anticipated benefit, even if life cannot be prolonged without treatment. This view was confirmed by the courts in the 1990 case of Re J [120] in which it was held that treatment need not be given when the patient 'suffered from physical disabilities so grave that his life would from *his point of view* be so intolerable' that if he were able to make a sound judgement, he would not choose treatment.

> Baby J
>
> Baby J was born at 27 weeks gestation and was severely brain damaged. He appeared to be blind and was expected to be deaf and unlikely ever to be able to speak or develop even limited intellectual abilities. Despite these disabilities he

was thought to feel pain in the same way as other babies. His life expectancy was uncertain and he required repeated, invasive procedures to keep him alive. The Court was asked to consider whether it would be lawful to withhold artificial ventilation in the event of his breathing stopping, even though he was not imminently dying, on the grounds that providing the treatment would not be in J's best interests. The judge held that antibiotics should be provided if J developed an infection but artificial ventilation could be withheld. He said that treatment need not be given when the patient 'suffered from physical disabilities so grave that his life would from *his point of view* be so intolerable' that if he were able to make a sound judgement, he would not choose treatment.

Re J [121]

Subsequent legal cases have discussed the relationship between 'intolerability' and best interests. The Court of Appeal in the Charlotte Wyatt case (see Section 48.1) said that 'intolerable to the child' should not be seen as additional to, but rather as one part of, the assessment of best interests. Summing up the intellectual process for judges in such cases, Lord Justice Wall said:

> 'The judge must decide what is in the child's best interests. In making that decision, the welfare of the child is paramount, and the judge must look at the question from the assumed point of view of the patient. There is a strong presumption in favour of a course of action which will prolong life, but that presumption is not irrebuttable. The term 'best interests' encompasses medical, emotional and other welfare issues. The court must conduct a balancing exercise in which all the relevant factors are weighed and a helpful way of undertaking this exercise is to draw up a balance sheet.' [122]

The 'balance sheet' approach is discussed in Section 22.2.

50.2. If a decision is reached to withhold or withdraw a particular treatment, it is essential to emphasise that this does not represent abandonment or 'giving up' on the child or young person but a realisation that continued treatment would not be in the patient's best interests.

It is important that parents recognise that it is the value of the *treatment* that is being assessed, not the value of the child or young person's life. Although the immediate goal may have shifted from seeking the benefits that arise from prolonging life to seeking those that arise from being comfortable and free from pain, the overall objective of providing benefit does not change. In the case of Charlotte Wyatt, Lord Justice Hedley specifically included securing a 'good death' as part of the assessment of best interests [123].

> *Summary – Assessing best interests*
>
> • *The key to decision making is the child or young person's best interests viewed from his or her own perspective*
> • *There is a presumption in favour of providing life-prolonging treatment but in each case the burdens of treatment must be weighed against the anticipated benefits*

51. Dealing with disagreement

51.1. The views of parents about whether to accept the treatment proposed by the health care team will usually be determinative unless the decision is contrary to the child or young person's best interests (see Section 9).

Where the parents hold strong views in favour of either withdrawing or continuing treatment, these, together with the reasons for their views, should be given serious consideration as part of the decision-making process. Where the parents make a decision that the health care team believes conflicts with the best interests of the child or young person, this should be explained to them and, where appropriate, a further clinical opinion should be offered. Frequently parents need to have reassurance that everything reasonable has been done and seeking an independent view from a different clinician can sometimes help to provide this. Speaking to someone with experience of the condition can also be helpful.

51.2. If agreement cannot be reached through discussion, it will be necessary to seek a court declaration about best interests.

In order to proceed with non-emergency treatment for a baby, child or young person who lacks capacity, consent must be obtained from either someone with parental responsibility or a court.

> *Summary – Dealing with disagreement*
>
> • *The views of the parents about whether to accept the treatment proposed by the health care team will usually be determinative unless they are contrary to the child or young person's best interests*
> • *If there is disagreement that cannot be resolved through discussion, the court should be asked to make a declaration*

Part 9 **Once a decision has been reached**

52. Keeping others informed

52.1. Health care proxies, welfare attorneys, deputies and those with parental responsibility for children should be kept informed of developments following their agreement to the withholding or withdrawal of treatment.

Once a course of action has been agreed, any health care proxy, welfare attorney, deputy or person with parental responsibility should be kept informed of all developments, including when and how the decision will be acted upon. Where there is any disagreement about the patient's best interests, immediate steps should be taken to resolve the problem.

52.2. Where there was no health care proxy, welfare attorney or deputy and the decision was made by the clinician in charge of the patient's care, those who were consulted in the process of assessing best interests should, wherever possible, be informed of the final decision and the reasons for it before it is implemented.

Providing an explanation for such decisions can help everyone concerned with the care of the patient to satisfy themselves that the proposed treatment would not provide a benefit to the patient and to come to terms with the situation. Where there is any disagreement about the patient's best interests, immediate steps should be taken to resolve the problem.

> *Summary – Keeping others informed*
>
> - *Those who were consulted in the process of assessing best interests, including health care proxies, welfare attorneys, court appointed deputies and those with parental responsibility should be informed of the final decision and the reasons for it*

53. Recording and reviewing the decision

53.1. The basis for the decision to withhold or withdraw life-prolonging treatment should be carefully documented in the patient's medical notes.

The clinician in charge of the patient's care should clearly record in the notes when and by whom the decision was made to withhold or withdraw a particular treatment, the basis on which the decision was reached, from whom information was received and the way in which it was used. Where treatment is refused by an adult with capacity, the patient should be asked to provide written confirmation of the refusal, if possible, and this should be held in the medical record. Where treatment is withheld or withdrawn in response to a valid advance decision refusing treatment, a copy of the advance decision should be held on the record together with a note of any further enquiries made about its validity. Where treatment is withdrawn on the basis of a decision by an appointed attorney or person with parental responsibility, this should be recorded in the notes together with a record of the discussion that took place. This should include giving details of any disagreement with the decision by members of the health care team or other people close to the patient and how any disagreement was resolved. If the decision was to withhold or withdraw artificial nutrition and hydration, details of the independent clinical review undertaken in compliance with GMC guidance (see Section 12.2) should be recorded in the medical record. Information about any other professional guidance consulted or advice sought should also be formally recorded.

Where patients are being cared for by their general practitioner in the community, such as in a nursing home, information should be recorded in both the general practitioner's notes and the nursing or medical notes held by the establishment within which the patient is being cared for.

53.2. Decisions to withhold or withdraw life-prolonging treatment should continue to be reviewed after implementation to take account of any change in circumstances.

It is often difficult to anticipate with certainty how a patient will respond once treatment is withdrawn. The patient's condition should be monitored after the withdrawal of treatment and decisions should be reviewed if there is a significant change in the circumstances. Those close to or representing the patient should be kept informed of developments and should be notified if the situation is not as expected. This is particularly important where there is a health care proxy, welfare attorney, deputy or person with parental responsibility who has the authority to make treatment decisions.

53.3. Decisions to withdraw or withhold life-prolonging treatment should be subject to review and audit.

Treatment providers and health care facilities have an ethical obligation to audit regularly their own patterns of decision making and compare them with wider trends. Health authorities should be encouraged to provide local guidelines addressing the decision-making process with a system of audit to ensure that the guidelines are being followed. Doctors must be able to demonstrate that their treatment recommendations comply with a responsible body of medical opinion and are in the best interests of each individual patient. Advice must be sought from professional bodies and the General Medical Council if anomalous patterns of decision making are identified in comparison with those of other clinicians or other similar facilities. Managers have an obligation to investigate promptly such trends in their facilities.

Those treating patients who lack the capacity to make or communicate decisions need to be aware of the dangers of decisions to withhold or withdraw treatment becoming routine. A constant awareness is needed that each individual decision must be carefully considered in order to ascertain whether the treatment would provide a net benefit to the particular patient. Doctors must be able to justify their decisions if called upon to do so.

Summary – Recording and reviewing the decision

- *The basis for the decision to withhold or withdraw treatment should be documented in the medical notes*
- *Decisions should be reviewed after implementation to take account of any changes in the circumstances*
- *Decisions should be subject to review and audit*

---

54. Providing support

54.1. Welfare attorneys and people with parental responsibility for children, who are responsible for making the decision to withhold or withdraw treatment, may be left with feelings of guilt and anxiety in addition to their bereavement. Similar feelings may also be experienced by relatives and friends who did not actually make the decision to withdraw treatment but who contributed to the assessment of best interests. It is important that such people are supported both before and after the decision has been made to withdraw or withhold life-prolonging treatment.

Providing support for the patient and those close to the patient to help them to come to terms with their bereavement is a routine part of caring for dying patients. Where the patient has died following a decision to withhold or withdraw life-prolonging treatment, however, the usual bereavement may be exacerbated by feelings of guilt or anxiety about whether the right decision was made and about the family's role in that decision. The family should be encouraged to discuss their concerns and, if appropriate, should be offered counselling.

54.2. The emotional and psychological burden on staff involved with withdrawing and withholding life-prolonging treatment should be recognised and adequate support mechanisms need to be available and easily accessible before, during and after decisions have been made.

Staff members' needs for support may easily be overlooked. Employing bodies and colleagues of those involved with making and carrying out these very difficult decisions need to be sensitive to the possibility of 'burnout' and to the need for adequate support mechanisms to be in place which are easily accessible to all staff. Staff at all levels should have access to counselling and support both within and outside the health care team. This is likely to be needed before, during and after the decision has been made and implemented.

Summary – Providing support

- *Those who have been involved with the decision to withhold or withdraw life-prolonging treatment may experience feelings of guilt, as well as bereavement and should be given emotional support*
- *The emotional burden on the staff involved with such decisions should be recognised and support provided*

---

55. Respecting patients' wishes after death

55.1. Part of the duty of care to dying patients is to take reasonable steps to facilitate any known wishes about, for example, organ and tissue donation, the handling of the body after death or any particular religious practices that were important to the patient.

Over 90% of the population express support for organ donation and with developments in non-heartbeating donation it is now possible for some solid organs to be donated following the controlled withdrawal of treatment; tissue donation may also be a possibility. Where treatment is withdrawn in circumstances that would enable organs and/or tissues to be donated, steps should be taken to determine the individual's wishes (including making enquiries with the organ donor register) and the transplant co-ordinator should be contacted at an early stage.

***

Summary – Respecting patients' wishes after death

- *Reasonable steps should be taken to facilitate the known wishes of the individual after death*

***

Appendix 1 **Useful addresses**

British Association for Parenteral and Enteral Nutrition (BAPEN), Secure Hold Business Centre, Studley Road, Redditch, Worcestershire B98 7LG. Tel: 01527 457 850, Fax: 01527 458 718
Website: www.bapen.org.uk

British Medical Association, BMA House, Tavistock Square, London WC1H 9JP. Tel: 020 7387 4499, Fax: 020 7383 6400
Email: info.public@bma.org.uk
Website: www.bma.org.uk

Children and Family Court Advisory and Support Service (CAFCASS) National Office, 8th Floor, South Quay Plaza 3, 189 Marsh Wall, London E14 9SH. Tel: 020 7510 7000, Fax: 020 7510 7001
Email: webenquiries@cafcass.gov.uk
Website: www.cafcass.gov.uk

Children and Family Court Advisory and Support Service (CAFCASS) Cymru, Llys y Delyn, 107–111 Cowbridge Road East, Cardiff CF11 9AG. Tel: 02920 647 979, Fax: 02920 398 540
Website: www.cafcass.gov.uk/cafcassCymru.htm

Health Professions Council, Park House, 184 Kennington Park Road, London SE11 4BU. Tel: 020 7582 0866, Fax: 020 7820 9684
Website: www.hpc-uk.org

Court of Protection, Archway Tower, 2 Junction Road, London N19 5SZ. Tel: 020 7664 7300, Fax: 020 7664 7168
Email: custserv@guardianship.gsi.gov.uk
Website: www.guardianship.gov.uk

Department for Constitutional Affairs, Selborne House, 54–60 Victoria Street, London SW1E 6QW. DX 117000 Selborne House. Tel: 020 7210 8500
Website: www.dca.gov.uk

Department of Health, Wellington House, 133–155 Waterloo Road, London SE1 8UG. Tel: 020 7972 2000
Website: www.dh.gov.uk

General Medical Council, Regent's Place, 350 Euston Road, London NW1 3JN. Tel: 020 7189 5404, Fax: 020 7189 5401
Email: standards@gmc-uk.org
Website: www.gmc-uk.org

Independent Mental Capacity Advocacy Service, Department of Health, Wellington House, 133 Waterloo Road, London SE1 8UG

Medical Defence Union, 230 Blackfriars Road, London SE1 8PJ. Tel: 020 7202 1500, Fax: 020 7202 1666
Website: www.the-mdu.com

Medical and Dental Defence Union of Scotland, Mackintosh House, 120 Blythswood Street, Glasgow G2 4EA. Tel: 0141 221 5858, Fax: 0141 228 1208
Website: www.mddus.com

Medical Protection Society, 33 Cavendish Square, London W1M 0PS. Tel: 020 7399 1300, Fax: 020 7399 1301
Website: www.mps-group.org

Mental Welfare Commission for Scotland, K Floor, Argyle House, 3 Lady Lawson Street, Edinburgh EH3 9SH. Tel: 0131 222 6111, Fax: 0131 222 6112
Email: enquiries@mwcscot.org.uk
Website: www.mwcscot.org.uk

Nursing & Midwifery Council (NMC), 23 Portland Place, London W1B 1PZ. Tel: 020 7637 7181, Fax: 020 7436 2924
Website: www.nmc-uk.org

Official Solicitor of the Supreme Court, 81 Chancery Lane, London WC2A 1DD. DX 0012 London/Chancery Lane. Tel: 020 7911 7127, Fax: 020 7911 7105
Email: enquiries@offsol.gsi.gov.uk
Website: www.officialsolicitor.gov.uk

Official Solicitor of the Supreme Court for Northern Ireland, Royal Courts of Justice, PO Box 410, Chichester Street, Belfast BT1 3JF. Tel: 028 9023 5111, Fax: 028 9031 3793
Email: officialsolicitorsoffice@courtsni.gov.uk
Website: www.courtsni.gov.uk

Office of the Public Guardian, Archway Tower, 2 Junction Road, London N19 5SZ. Tel: 0845 330 2900, Fax: 0870 739 5780
Email: custserv@guardianship.gsi.gov.uk
Website: www.guardianship.gov.uk

Office of the Public Guardian, Scotland, Hadrian House, Callendar Business Park, Callendar Road, Falkirk FK1 1XR. DX 550360 FALKIRK 3. Tel: 01324 678 300, Fax: 01324 678 301
Email: opg@scotcourts.org.uk
Website: www.publicguardian-scotland.gov.uk

Patients Association, PO Box 935, Harrow, Middlesex HA1 3YJ. Tel: 020 8423 9111, Fax: 020 8423 9119
Email: mailbox@patients-association.com
Website: www.patients-association.org.uk

Resuscitation Council (UK), 5th Floor, Tavistock House North, Tavistock Square, London WC1H 9HR. Tel: 020 7388 4678, Fax: 020 7383 0773
Email: enquiries@resus.org.uk
Website: www.resus.org.uk

Royal College of General Practitioners, 14 Princes Gate, Hyde Park, London SW7 1PU. Tel: 020 7581 3232, Fax: 020 7225 3047
Email: info@rcgp.org.uk
Website: www.rcgp.org.uk

Royal College of Nursing, 20 Cavendish Square, London W1M 0AB. Tel: 020 7409 3333, Fax: 020 7647 3435
Website: www.rcn.org.uk

Royal College of Paediatrics and Child Health, 50 Hallam Street, London W1W 6DE. Tel: 020 7307 5600, Fax: 020 7307 5601
Email: enquiries@rcpch.ac.uk
Website: www.rcpch.ac.uk

Royal College of Physicians, 11 St Andrew's Place, London NW1 4LE. Tel: 020 7935 1174, Fax: 020 7487 5218
Website: www.rcplondon.ac.uk

Royal College of Physicians and Surgeons of Glasgow, 232–242 St Vincent Street, Glasgow G2 5RJ. Tel: 0141 221 6072, Fax: 0141 221 1804
Website: www.rcpsglasg.ac.uk

Royal College of Physicians of Edinburgh, 9 Queen Street, Edinburgh EH2 1JQ. Tel: 0131 225 7324, Fax: 0131 220 3939
Website: www.rcpe.ac.uk

Royal College of Surgeons of Edinburgh, Nicolson Street, Edinburgh EH8 9DW. Tel: 0131 527 1600, Fax: 0131 557 6406
Email: information@rcsed.ac.uk
Website: www.rcsed.ac.uk

Royal College of Surgeons of England, 35–43 Lincoln's Inn Fields, London WC2A 3PE. Tel: 020 7405 3474, Fax: 020 7831 9438
Website: www.rcseng.ac.uk

References

1. R (on the application of Burke) v General Medical Council [2005] 2 FLR 1223 at 69.
2. General Medical Council (2002). *Withholding and Withdrawing Life-prolonging Treatments: Good Practice in Decision-making*. GMC, London.
3. Royal College of Paediatrics and Child Health (1997). *Withholding or Withdrawing Life Saving Treatment in Children. A Framework for Practice*. RCPCH, London.
4. Scottish Executive (2002). *Adults with Incapacity (Scotland) Act 2000 Code of Practice for Persons Authorised to Carry Out Medical Treatment or Research under Part 5 of the Act. SE/2002/73*. Scottish Executive, Edinburgh.
5. Department for Constitutional Affairs (2007). *Mental Capacity Act 2005 Code of Practice*. DCA, London.
6. Mental Capacity Act 2005 s.3(1); Re MB (medical treatment) [1997] 2 FLR No 3.
7. Jackson E (2006). *Medical Law. Text, Cases and Materials*. Oxford University Press, Oxford, pp. 201–3.
8. R (on the application of Burke) v General Medical Council [2005] Op cit.
9. Ibid.
10. Ibid at 50.
11. Re R (adult: medical treatment) [1996] 2 FLR 99.
12. Re J (a minor) (wardship: medical treatment) [1990] 3 All ER 930 at 55.
13. Re R (adult: medical treatment) [1996] Op cit.
14. Salek S, Finlay IG (2004). The use of quality of life instruments in palliative care. *European Journal of Palliative Care* 9(2): 52–6; Salek S (1999). *Compendium of Quality of Life Instruments*. Wiley, Chichester.
15. R (on the application of Burke) v General Medical Council [2005] Op cit at 53.
16. See, for example: NHS End of Life Care Programme (2006). *Progress Report, March 2006*. Department of Health, London.
17. Mental Capacity Act 2005 s.4(6).
18. R (on the application of Burke) v General Medical Council [2005] Op cit at 33.
19. See British Medical Association (2004). *Medical Ethics Today – The BMA's Handbook of Ethics and Law*, 2nd edition. BMJ Books, London, pp. 747–8.
20. Jackson E (2006). *Medical Law. Text, Cases and Materials*. Op cit, pp. 206–9.
21. For more specific guidance on the provision and withdrawal of artificial nutrition and hydration, see British Association for Parenteral and Enteral Nutrition (BAPEN) (1998). *Ethical and Legal Aspects of Clinical Hydration and Nutritional Support*. BAPEN, London.
22. Treloar A, Howard P (1998). Tube feeding: medical treatment or basic care? *Catholic Medical Quarterly* August:5–7.

23. General Medical Council (2002). *Withholding and Withdrawing Life-prolonging Treatments: Good Practice in Decision-making.* Op cit, para 81.
24. Airedale NHS Trust v Bland [1993] 1 All ER 821.
25. Ibid.
26. See, for example, Frenchay Healthcare NHS Trust v S [1994] 1 WLR 601; Re D (medical treatment) [1998] 1 FLR 411.
27. Law Hospital NHS Trust v Lord Advocate (1996) SLT 848.
28. General Medical Council (2002). *Withholding and Withdrawing Life-prolonging Treatments: Good Practice in Decision-Making.* Op cit, para 81.
29. Baines M, Sykes NP (2000). Symptom management and palliative care. In: Evans JG, Williams TF, Beattie BL, Michel JP, Wilcock GK (eds). *Oxford Textbook of Geriatric Medicine,* 2nd edition. Oxford University Press, Oxford, pp. 1113–26.
30. R v Woollin [1998] 4 All ER 103.
31. NHS Trust A v M; NHS Trust B v H [2001] 1 All ER 801.
32. Airedale NHS Trust v Bland [1993] Op cit.
33. See, for example, Re J (a minor) (child in care: medical treatment) [1992] 3 WLR 507.
34. Portsmouth NHS Trust v Wyatt, 21 October 2005 (unreported); Locke D. *Children and Patients Without Legal Capacity and Medical Treatment: The Law after the Burke and Charlotte Wyatt Cases.* Mills & Reeve, Birmingham.
35. R (on the application of Burke) v General Medical Council [2005] Op cit at 40.
36. See R v North West Lancashire Health Authority, ex parte A, D & G [2000] 1 WLR 977; R (on the application of K) v West London Mental Health Trust [2006] 1 WLR 1865.
37. Joint Committee on Human Rights (2004). *Joint Committee on Human Rights – Seventh Report. The Meaning of Public Authority under the Human Rights Act. Session 2003–04.* The Stationery Office, London.
38. Human Rights Act 1998 s.6(6).
39. Vo v France (2005) 40 EHRR 12.
40. NHS Trust A v M; NHS Trust B v H [2001] Op cit at 49.
41. R (on the application of Burke) v General Medical Council [2004] 2 FLR 1121 at 145.
42. A National Health Service Trust v D & Ors [2000] 2 FLR 677.
43. General Medical Council (2002). *Withholding and Withdrawing Life-prolonging Treatments: Good Practice in Decision-making.* Op cit, para 25.
44. NHS Trust v (1) S (2) DG (3) SG [2003] Lloyd's Rep Med 137 at 49.
45. Ibid.
46. R (on the application of Burke) v General Medical Council [2004] Op cit at 35.
47. See also Re A (male sterilisation) [2001] FLR 549.
48. An NHS Trust v MB [2006] Fam Law 445 at 60.
49. British Medical Association, Resuscitation Council (UK), Royal College of Nursing (2002). *Decisions Relating to Cardiopulmonary Resuscitation.* BMA, London.
50. Re MB (medial treatment) [1997] 2 FLR 3.
51. Re B (adult: refusal of medical treatment) [2002] 2 All ER 449.

52. Ibid.
53. St George's Healthcare National Health Service Trust v S (No 2): R v Louize Collins & Ors, Ex Parte S (No 2) [1998] 3 WLR 936. See also Department of Health (1999). *Consent to Treatment – Summary of Legal Rulings, HSC 1999/031.* DH, London.
54. St George's Healthcare National Health Service Trust v S (No 2): R v Louize Collins & Ors, Ex Parte S (No 2) Op cit.
55. Re B (adult: refusal of medical treatment) [2002] Op cit.
56. British Medical Association (2007). *The Mental Capacity Act 2005: Guidance for Health Professionals.* BMA, London.
57. Mental Capacity Act 2005 s.1.
58. Department for Constitutional Affairs (2007). *Mental Capacity Act 2005 Code of Practice.* Op cit, chapter 5.
59. Mental Capacity Act 2005 s.24–26.
60. Department for Constitutional Affairs (2007). *Mental Capacity Act 2005 Code of Practice.* Op cit, chapter 9.
61. Mental Capacity Act 2005 s.25(2).
62. Mental Capacity Act 2005 s.25(4).
63. Re T (adult: refusal of medical treatment) [1992] 4 All ER 649. See also HE v A NHS Trust [2003] 2 FLR 408; X NHS Trust v T (adult: refusal of medical treatment) [2005] 1 All ER 387.
64. Re AK (medical treatment: consent) [2001] 1 FLR 129.
65. Department for Constitutional Affairs (2007). *Mental Capacity Act 2005 Code of Practice.* Op cit, chapter 5.
66. The Mental Capacity Act 2005 (Independent Mental Capacity Advocates) (General) Regulations 2006. SI 2006 No 1832: para 4(2).
67. Lennard-Jones JE (1999). Giving or withholding fluids and nutrients: ethical and legal aspects. *Journal of the Royal College of Physicians of London* **33**(1): 39–45.
68. W Healthcare NHS Trust v H [2005] 1 WLR 834.
69. Ibid.
70. British Medical Association (2002). *Medical Treatment for Adults with Incapacity. Guidance on Ethical and Medico-legal Issues in Scotland,* 2nd edition. BMA, London.
71. Scottish Executive (2002). *Adults with Incapacity (Scotland) Act 2000 Code of Practice for Persons Authorised to Carry Out Medical Treatment or Research under Part 5 of the Act. SE/2002/73.* Op cit, para 2.29.
72. See, for example: Airedale NHS Trust v Bland [1993] Op cit; Re T (adult: refusal of medical treatment) [1992] Op cit; Re C (adult: refusal of treatment) [1994] 1 WLR 290.
73. Re T (adult: refusal of medical treatment) [1992] Op cit.
74. Re C (adult: refusal of treatment) [1994] Op cit.
75. Ibid.
76. Law Hospital NHS Trust v Lord Advocate (1996) Op cit.

77. See, for example: Airedale NHS Trust v Bland [1993] Op cit; Re T (adult: refusal of treatment) [1992] Op cit; Re C (adult: refusal of medical treatment) [1994] Op cit.
78. Re F (mental patient: sterilisation) sub nom F v West Berkshire Health Authority [1989] 2 All ER 545.
79. Ibid.
80. Mental Capacity Act 2005 s.3(1); Re MB (medical treatment) [1997] Op cit.
81. See, for example, Secker AB, Meier DA, Mulvihill MPH, Paris BEC (1991). Substituted judgment: how accurate are proxy predictions? *Annals of Internal Medicine* **115**(2):92–8; Gerety MB, Chiodo LK, Kanten DN, Tuley MR, Cornell JE (1993). Medical treatment preferences of nursing home residents: relationship to function and concordance with surrogate decision-makers. *Journal of the American Geriatrics Society* **41**:953–60; Emanuel EJ, Emanuel LL (1992). Proxy decision making for incompetent patients: an ethical and empirical analysis. *Journal of the American Medical Association* **267**:2067–71.
82. Gillick v West Norfolk and Wisbech Area Health Authority [1986] AC 122; R (on the application of Axon) v Secretary of State for Health [2006] 2 WLR 1130.
83. Gillick v West Norfolk and Wisbech Area Health Authority [1986] Op cit.
84. Ibid.
85. Re R (a minor) [1991] 4 All ER 177.
86. Re W (a minor) (medical treatment) [1992] 4 All ER 649.
87. Re P (medical treatment: best interests) [2004] 2 FLR 1117 at 9.
88. Ibid.
89. Age of Legal Capacity (Scotland) Act 1991 s.1(1)(b) and 2(4).
90. Children (Scotland) Act 1995 s.16(2).
91. Houston (applicant) (1996) 32 BMLR 93.
92. Re MB (medical treatment) [1997] Op cit.
93. British Medical Association (2001). *Consent, Rights and Choices in Health Care for Children and Young People.* BMJ Books, London.
94. National Institute for Health and Clinical Excellence (NICE) (2005). *Improving Outcomes in Child and Adolescent Cancer Services. The Evidence Review.* NICE, London, Appendix D: Consultation with children with cancer, their siblings and parents for the NICE child and adolescent cancer service guidelines.
95. Children Act 1989 s.1(3); Children (Scotland) Act 1995 s.6(1) and s.16(2); UN Convention on the Rights of the Child 1989 (Article 12). See also Human Rights Act 1998 s 1 and schedule 1, Articles 8 and 10.
96. Royal College of Nursing (2003). *Restraining, Holding Still and Containing Children: Guidance for Good Practice*, 2nd edition. RCN, London.
97. Royal College of Paediatrics and Child Health (1997). *Withholding or Withdrawing Life Saving Treatment in Children.* Op cit.
98. For further information see British Medical Association (2006). *Parental Responsibility. Guidance from the BMA's Ethics Department.* BMA, London.
99. Civil Partnership Act 2004.
100. Children Act 1989 s.1(3).

101. Children (Scotland) Act 1995 s.11(7).
102. Children (Northern Ireland) Order 1995 art 3(1).
103. Re C (medical treatment) [1998] 1 FLR 384.
104. Ibid.
105. An NHS Trust v MB [2006] Op cit.
106. Ibid.
107. Re T (a minor) (wardship: medical treatment); sub nom Re C (a minor) (parents' consent to surgery) [1997] 1 All ER 906.
108. Re C (welfare of child: immunisation) [2003] 2 FLR 1095.
109. Re T (a minor) (wardship: medical treatment); sub nom Re C (a minor) (parents' consent to surgery) [1997] Op cit.
110. Glass v United Kingdom (2004) (application no. 61827/00).
111. Nelson LJ et al. (1995). Forgoing medically provided nutrition and hydration in pediatric patients. *Journal of Law, Medicine and Ethics* **23**:33–46.
112. Portsmouth NHS Trust v Wyatt [2005] 1 FLR 21.
113. Ibid.
114. Portsmouth NHS Trust v Wyatt [2005] EWHC 117.
115. Portsmouth NHS Trust v Wyatt [2005] 2 FLR 480.
116. Portsmouth NHS Trust v Wyatt [2006] 1 FLR 554.
117. Portsmouth NHS Trust v Wyatt, 21 October 2005 (unreported).
118. Portsmouth NHS Trust v Wyatt [2006] Fam Law 359.
119. Portsmouth NHS Trust v Wyatt [2005] 1 FLR 21.
120. Re J (a minor) (wardship: medical treatment) [1990] Op cit.
121. Ibid.
122. Portsmouth NHS Trust v Wyatt [2006] 1 FLR 554 at 87.
123. Portsmouth NHS Trust v Wyatt [2005] 1 FLR 21.

Index

acute renal failure, 29
Adults with Incapacity Act, 26, 62–5, 67, 81
advance decisions about medical treatment,
    46–7
  England and Wales, 52–6
  Northern Ireland, 69
  refusal of life-prolonging treatment, 52–5,
    64–7, 85, 87
  request for life-prolonging treatment, 56,
    67, 85, 89
  Scotland, 63–7
Age of Legal Capacity Act, 89–90
Airedale NHS Trust v. Bland, 16–17, 19
Alzheimer's disease, 54
amputation, 66
An NHS Trust v. MB, 100
ANH. *See* artificial nutrition and hydration
    (ANH)
anorexia nervosa, 86
antibiotics, 5
artificial nutrition and hydration (ANH), 5,
    10–11, 15–18
  provision of, 6–7, 44
  refusal of, 46
  request for, 85, 89
  separate assessment of, 15–16
  withholding or withdrawal of, 7, 16, 58–62,
    68–69, 71–2, 85
artificial ventilation, 5, 41, 44, 99
autism, 29
AV fistula, 29–30
awareness of patient, 11, 77–78

balance sheet approach, 34–5
basic care, 15–18, 42, 53
basic human rights, infringement of, 12
benefit of life-prolonging treatment, 10–12,
    19, 34, 63, 77–9, 85. *See also* best
    interests of patient
best interests of patient, 51–2, 85–6, 96.
    See also benefit of life-prolonging
    treatment

assessment of, 12–14, 20, 30, 34–5, 40,
    57–9, 74–80, 106–7
  disagreements about, 20, 52, 67–8, 80–81,
    97, 99–102
bilateral renal dysplasia, 29
biliary atresia, 100
Bland, Tony, 16–17, 19, 61
Bolam test, 14, 35
brain, malformation of, 8–9
Brown, Sir Stephen, 9
Burke v. General Medical Council (GMC), 6–7,
    14, 20, 21, 25–6, 30, 44, 59
Burke, Oliver Leslie, 6–7. See also *Burke v.
    General Medical Council (GMC)*
Butler-Sloss, Lady Justice, 25, 29–30

Caesarean section, 45–6
capacity. *See also* capacity, lack of
  adults with, 43–8
  assessment of, 5–7, 91–2
  legal presumption of, 43, 47, 51, 54, 72,
    84
  varying levels of, 72–3
  young people with, 83–95
capacity, lack of. *See also* capacity
  adults with, 50–81
  assessment of, 5–6
  children and young people with,
    96–108
cardiac arrest, 38
cardiopulmonary resuscitation, 5, 38
cavernoma, 45
cerebellar ataxia with peripheral neuropathy,
    6–7
cerebral palsy, 8–9
chemotherapy, 5
Children Act, 89, 98–9
Coleridge, Justice, 59–60
communication. *See* decision making,
    communication and information for
confidentiality, 32–3, 76–7
conscientious objection, 20–21, 45

123